THE
Sepsis
Cure

THE Sepsis Cure

WILLIAM NORBERG, MD

Published by Sepaalbu LLC
www.TNSrx-Sepsis.com

ISBN (paperback): 979-8-9884934-0-2
ISBN (ebook): 979-8-9884934-1-9

Book design and production by www.AuthorSuccess.com

Printed in the United States of America

Contents

DISCLAIMER

All information has been accepted using a standard methodology for medical decision-making, Reasonable Medical Certainty.

Reasonable Medical Certainty (RMC) is the level of review that is commonly used in medical practice.

Determining the benefits versus the risks results in a decision that treatment is more likely to be helpful.

This is the level of decision-making the physicians use when providing direct patient care.

RMC is the established standard that was used during the patient care cited and used throughout this book.

This decision level ranges from "won't hurt" to "avoid as unlikely to help and likely to hurt." This decision process incorporates the known facts that can be directly applied to the care, but the expansion of this decision must also include the patient, the disease, and the physician.

Physicians and caregivers who access the information are held to the standard of RMC. No formulas, suggestions, or implications can in any way be used directly for patient care. No legal or medical liability can be inferred or in any way imply a responsibility for any situation that could result. Clinical decision-making remains the sole responsibility of the treating physician.

This book includes generally available medical research data and other scientific presentations, but no claim or inference is made that this is a comprehensive review. Readily available medical literature from open sites have been reviewed. Data and information from conferences and meetings that were supportive was included. Again, the low level requirement of RMC was the standard applied.

It is anticipated some controversy will be generated by this book, as the scientific evidence leaves large holes that are now bridged with assumptions. Many controversies will be resolved by more and better data. No implication or claim is ever made about the comprehensive and thoroughness of the background research.

Many more articles and valuable contributions will be found as time passes. Conflicting and confounding information is to be anticipated. These new items should add to the overall knowledge base.

No prescription for treatment of any patient for any disease or condition are presented in this book.

In summary, physicians utilizing information presented in this book will get the greatest benefit when each individual physician applies his personal medical knowledge and uses the RMC standard that every physician has developed.

Presented for your benefit, your clinical care colleague,

William J Norberg MD

Introduction

I was tired of watching children die.

After spending decades as a pediatric cardiologist, I had to see too many families grieve the loss of the light in their world. One of the most common causes of their demise was not the issues with their heart, but the resulting sepsis that developed after their treatment. But while those who were researching cures were looking in one direction, I used my experience and knowledge to try something new and innovative ... something that actually worked!

Sepsis is a term heard directly related to very ill or recently deceased people. Yet our understanding of sepsis is poor, no matter what your education level.

The "official" definition is **Sepsis is a life-threatening organ dysfunction caused by dysregulated host response to disease.** However, sepsis is a complex problem and exists without a simple definition. But it is my hope that after reading this book, you will not only fully understand just what sepsis is, but also that it does NOT have to be a death sentence.

To help you fully understand, I have included patient care stories and explanations of the developing role of the specialty of Critical Care Medicine. These heartwrenching patient care experiences provided the strong incentive for me to find the cause of and a cure for sepsis.

The book introduces the reader to current limitations of modern medicine and emphasizes the need for a cure. Frustrated by years of research that failed to provide clear answers, I will explain the complex steps that were involved in the search through the years that ultimately led me to develop The Norberg Solution (TNS), the cure for sepsis, along with the barriers that had to be overcome along the way.

The path to getting TNS to the patient is almost as much of a miracle as the actual miracle treatment itself.

There never has been another story like this.

Learn about this miracle medication that could truly save your or your loved one's life.

TNS is my gift to the world, and it is my honor to make this contribution to medicine.

William Norberg MD

CHAPTER ONE

The Problems with Sepsis Today

Sadness resolves only with the passage of time. So many details are lost over the years, but the emotions of the moment remain. As each patient's case is reviewed here, the memories return with total recall and the stress and anxiety of that time all return rapidly and at full force. Too many times only the sadness and the failure remain.

This sadness of personal loss is the saga of sepsis. This terrible disease continues to beat us down.

This book tells the stories of Critical Care from clinical cases and the scientific world.

Sepsis was the impetus for creating the intensive and critical care specialties to try to help mitigate the severe medical problems it caused. While the development of these specialties has improved the quality of patient care, the answer to stopping sepsis has eluded medical professionals to this day, despite intensive and continuous efforts to do so.

The girl in this first case study was an index critical care patient, cared for at the onset of critical care development. Her outcome is intimately associated with the recognition of sepsis as a killer disease of all humanity.

Case 1. The Onset of the Critical Care Specialty

A seventeen-year-old girl was brought to the hospital with progressive respiratory failure and shock. She had only been sick for three days but was getting progressively worse. No one could figure out why she was sick and the hospital she had been taken to was unable to give her the care that she needed, but they did recognize that she was critically ill. They transferred her to another medical facility that had more resources to care for her.

The hospital-to-hospital transfer was routinely accepted, but the people, the hospital, the procedures, and all the things that were familiar to the patient and her family completely changed with the transfer. In this new setting, the family met many new people with confusing names and titles. Even though each person was an essential part of the Pediatric Intensive Care Unit (PICU) team, the girl's family was having a hard time adjusting to the change during this difficult and frightening time.

A tertiary care Pediatric Intensive Care Unit (PICU) has a unique setting. The patient bed is the same as you would find in any hospital room, but the attached wires lead to the monitor with an almost continuously beeping vital sign monitor. The Intensive Care Unit nursing desk is in direct view of the nursing station to monitor the patient directly. The whole Unit carries a tense sense of urgency; a feeling that "this is an emergency, and all things need to be addressed now!"

When she arrived, the girl was quite frightened and very anxious. She was breathing rapidly with some difficulty, despite a nasal oxygen cannula in place. Her lips were blue, her hands were white. Her pale face and her eyes projected the fear she was obviously feeling, which rubbed off on everyone she came into contact with.

Through her extreme fear and anxiety, she politely said to each person on the team, "Doctor promise me that you won't let me die."

Their response was an automatic, "We will take good care of you."

Translation: *Oh, how we wish we could promise that you will not die. But we do not control that decision.*

The situation was grim. Her blood pressure was low and her pulse is rapid and thready. The blood was circulating so slowly through her body that the return of any color (perfusion) to her hands was so slow that it was nearly nonexistent. She had an abnormally rapid heart rate and could only breathe with rapid grunts that did not provide enough air to her lungs. She needed help immediately!

The crisis response team quickly gave her intravenous fluids (Normal saline bolus of 20 ml per kilogram) at the maximum rate and ventilatory support from the beside ventilator. They kept the tools needed to place an endotracheal tube for respiratory control within reach.

"We are going to give you some medicine to let you sleep while we do some things," the doctors told her. "Everything will be okay."

But the odds of that being the case were poor, with a more than 69 percent probability of death from this terrible problem of septic shock. In fact, those were the last conscious words that the girl ever heard.

They did their very best, sedating her to place the endotracheal tube to provide better ventilation. The ventilator's moderate pressure improved her color to pink and the bolus of fluid improved perfusion so that her blood pressure returned to a low normal measurement, but was kept in an induced coma to help her body to heal.

However, everything went downhill from then. Her respiratory status steadily worsened, and her breathing became more labored, even with the ventilator. Her chest x-ray showed progressively increasing extensive pulmonary infiltrations.

Her blood pressure fell, she went into shock, and they gave her more fluids. This continued in a downward spiral cycle, with each round of treatment having less and less of a positive effect. All known interventions and support were in use, and urgent discussions ensued to search for any additional treatment options, but no answers were ever found.

Despite the best efforts of everyone on the team, her situation steadily got worse and worse and worse until finally, she deteriorated to a state of refractory pulmonary failure with severe hypoxia and acidosis, leading to cardiac arrest and could not be resuscitated.

This post death care review was incredibly difficult for all her caregivers. Despite our best efforts, we could not keep our promise to her; we had lied to her. We could not keep her from dying! Sepsis has won this round.

This was a young woman from a good and caring family, on the cusp of a wonderful future. She was smart, well on her way to becoming class Valedictorian, elected to be the Homecoming Queen, a member of the cheerleading squad, and had a life full of many more accomplishments. Her successful life only made her loss even worse.

Her death, like every patient's death, was such a huge and total loss to everyone involved with her care. There were no words that could comfort everyone who cared for her. The intensive care unit was very quiet that day.

The death review affirmed that all the known treatment modalities and interventions were performed at the correct time and properly applied. Good clinical care had been provided by all. Everything medically possible had been done well, but it just wasn't enough.

This was an initial case of septic shock related to a presumed primary pulmonary infection, early in the recognition of the magnitude of septic shock as a disease.

Her sepsis illness had continued to progress without response to all available medical interventions. Sepsis had no known treatment then and that is still the case to this day.

Our conclusion of this case review was that we had done as much as could be done and there were no further treatment options.

I decided right then and there that an answer to sepsis must be found! There must be something better that we can do!

Thus began the long and difficult search to **find the cure for sepsis**.

This book is the story of this clinician's lifetime search for a cause and treatment of sepsis.

This investigation of the cause and treatment of sepsis was generated by many patient deaths occurring in every doctor's experience treating sepsis: death despite best medical efforts. These continuing disasters were the basis for the establishment of this new medical specialty.

The medical cases presented in this book are true patient care stories. The need for a sepsis cure was repeatedly reinforced by the pain caused by each patient's death. There are too many stories of terrible medical losses from sepsis, and these stories continue to this day.

The Worst Disease of Humanity

Sepsis was defined in 2016 **as a life-threatening organ dysfunction caused by a deregulated host response to infection.**[1] This "precise" definition remains difficult to understand and particularly more difficult to explain to everyone.

Sepsis is difficult to define, even for those with advanced medical knowledge.

The June 2022 *Critical Care Medicine* journal published two different articles, and each article had a slightly different definition of sepsis but with essentially the same physiologic result, clearly showing the persistent difficulty with sepsis as a definition in addition to sepsis as a disease.

Sepsis appears to have its origin in the inflammatory response process of the body to infection or injury. These injuries include infection as the most recognized cause, but so many other causes also incite the inflammatory cascade. These other etiologies will likely be included in the sepsis classification in the future.

This inflammatory cascade proceeds at times to get out of control, become destructive, and then causing damage to the organs and organ systems of the body. This physiologic process of deterioration eventually progresses to death. This clinically is accepted as sepsis and septic shock.

The sepsis syndrome is a pattern of severe cellular injuries from the activation of this cytokine cascade (inflammatory response). The organ dysfunction leads to organ failure and eventually organ death. Sepsis is at its end phase; a mechanism of individual organ and cellular death that causes the host organism to die. Sepsis may be the process of death for the human organism.

Sepsis has always been linked primarily to bacterial infections. Sepsis is an extremely variable disease in its clinical presentation, leading to confusion during its presentation and difficulty even determining when the syndrome actually starts. The problem when defining sepsis with such a narrow description of the term is that the word "sepsis" remains inadequate to include all situations.

Ignaz Semmelweis (discussed later), who first recognized the peri-childbirth infections and the deaths of those women who suffered from them, remarked that there were large differences from case to case, but in the end all patients died.

These similarities but differences in disease presentation still create problems when exact pathological diagnoses are needed for clinical applications and statistical analysis.

Even the documentation of sepsis incidence across the world is very difficult to quantify. So many deaths are associated with another diagnosis named as the primary disease. These deaths are often attributed to the primary disease with sepsis as the terminal factor in the death, but sepsis is never recorded.

The sepsis diagnosis may not be addressed when the final primary medical cause of death is entered into the official database, where secondary diagnosis may or may not be recorded or counted. In general, the data is not "clean," as clinical definitions are all locally applied.

In 2017, the estimated number of cases due to sepsis was 44.9 million worldwide. Statistical reports of sepsis vary widely but all are very grim. This does not seem to vary much over the years.

Sepsis continues to be the worst disease of humanity. Sepsis has killed billions of people from antiquity to the present day. While the exact number of people dying of sepsis is difficult to obtain, it is obvious that the number is unbelievably large and much greater than any other disease.

By any measure, sepsis has a huge impact on human survival.

Sepsis is and always has been the greatest single killer of humanity. This ranking never changes; the statistics have wide ranges with variable sensitivity.

During the Covid-19 pandemic, this diagnostic dilemma was even worse. Was it sepsis or Covid? The reality was that sepsis was a manifestation of the pathophysiology of the Covid virus.

The recognition of the frequency and severity of the clinical problem supports the intensive search for drugs, chemicals, antibodies, or anything that would make a change in the treatment of patients with sepsis. Little has been found to this day, despite huge expenditures and a strong and dedicated effort.

Diseases leading to death have always been disruptive in every human social grouping. Keeping the people that we love alive and returning that individual person to a functional life has been an eternal goal of healers throughout human existence.

Every civilization has been afflicted by sepsis, and all have searched for a cure for anything that caused death.

Search for a Cure

My treatment was developed using a clinically-focused research approach using observations leading directly to conclusions. The medical care study of sepsis presented here used intense observation of sick patients within an intensive care setting. Each child presented with a similar but unique course of illness. The in-depth knowledge of the problems and complications of sepsis was derived from the focused observation during the care of each patient. Every patient added to the experience base, whatever the medical outcome.

Additional knowledge about sepsis was derived from failed clinical trials and the limited clinical response to new medical therapies and different medications. These treatment experiences built a knowledge base about sepsis, and that extensive scientific knowledge has been combined with the laboratory research work of countless people to build a huge database.

This data plus patient-based knowledge eventually became the key to developing a new therapy for sepsis. This new inflammatory response perspective originated from the bedside assessment of patient care problems with sepsis. This new and different understanding of the inflammatory cascade is also supported by scientific medical literature in variable degrees of concordance.

The new theory of inflammatory disease in its original presentation is here in this book. This new inflammatory disease hypothesis resulted from the integration of bedside observations and scientific research results.

This new concept of the inflammatory process in sepsis has never been discussed or presented at any scientific conference. Open presentation was compromised by the Covid pandemic causing the shutdown of conferences. The severe disruption of society in the attempts to minimize the deaths from the Covid-19 pandemic was not free.

Direct observation is the classic method of clinical medical research. Observed and documented manifestations of the patient's disease have been the basis of many original medical discoveries throughout the centuries.

This report of clinical application in the treatment of patients uses direct observation and case studies. These studies are limited by numbers and individual variability. These case reports continue to have an undeniably important role in medical research.

This pattern of investigation provides the weakest form of scientific data. The individual variability and the inability to recreate the exact situation again limits confidence. It is nearly impossible to control all the variables to recreate equivalent situations.

Modern scientific studies generally prefer identical situation comparisons. The gold standard is the double-blinded randomly assigned matched groups for best comparison of end results of controlled treatments. However, this double-blinded random methodology cannot be applied to this report's database.

Recently computerized tools for statistical data analysis were added to the armamentarium of medicines, equipment, and techniques available to the medical researchers and practitioners to further refine the conclusions. Valid interpretation of the computerized data presented in many published articles lead to identification of very subtle aberrancies have been facilitated by computer analysis. These observations show a beneficial impact hopefully leading to better clinical results. Current methods of analysis are used to improve the "quality" of the data and conclusions provided.

While treating patients who were suffering from sepsis, I explored the possibility primarily through such observations that inflammation could be a major part of sepsis. The clinical observation of dramatic modification of their disease process by the application of a newly created modified protein product brought a whole new focus to the treatment of sepsis.

The discovery of this new Inflammatory theory was not an orphan project. It was supported by the whole body of scientific research and modern biochemical pathophysiologic accomplishments. This is an integration of all information available formulated to come to a new conclusion.

Historically all the medical interventions applied toward control of sepsis have failed to reverse the illness. Nothing has been found to support the capacity of afflicted patients fighting sepsis to help alter the course of sepsis.

The natural course of sepsis illness is progressions in each patient to the predetermined end. Why some patients survive, and other patients do not, remains a medical mystery.

Covid-19 is, in our world today, a s pandemic presentation. For all those patients who develop the sepsis complication, medical science still has no effective medical treatment. Those patients who develop sepsis syndrome with Covid still have a random but very high mortality rate.

Specific beneficial interventions to control the virus at its inception are developing to prevent or modify the Covid disease, but still there remains *no specific medical treatment* for the disease of Covid-19 sepsis once the sepsis syndrome has begun.

Supportive organ function techniques are frequently applied, and with an organ failure bridge some patients are able to muster up enough intrinsic healing to make up their own cure. Most of these answers about healing are still awaiting discovery.

The therapeutic plan today is the same as always: **HOPE** you do not get the disease, and if that avoidance plan fails, **HOPE** you will not get sick enough to die.

No popular medical interventions alter the outcome.

Better and more complex supportive measures are used to support the patient through the crisis of organ or multiorgan failure.

Organ substitution techniques are available and are being used more frequently. These interventions work to allow more time for spontaneous recovery and keep the afflicted from dying until they can do it themselves.

For this pandemic, the vaccination program, the antibody infusion methodology, and the newly created antivirals new to Covid-19 do provide a benefit for many patients.

If you do not get the disease, you will not die of that disease.

The established medical support measures are known and are applied for prevention and treatments of early Covid and for many other diseases. These measures have limited treatment benefits and seem to work best when applied early. Antibody infusions primarily are related to prevention. The anti-viral medications cause modification of the early infection before the establishment of the viral reduplication process gets started and spreads throughout the entire body, causing the illness.

The history of human disease has been significantly altered by some medical achievements that are related to our essential disease management approach. These breakthrough accomplishments are even more outstanding considering the primitive state of the scientific art at that time, the very limited resources available, and the scarcity of helpful scientific data.

The current huge scientific body of knowledge today had a major supporting role that facilitated the creation of this new dynamic inflammatory cascade description. This same scientific information supported the development of the breakthrough medical product that changed the course of sepsis. These clinical observations were made and fully supported by the academic awareness of the other works in this area.

The current clinical medical investigations are a process of an analysis of a large number of cases resulting in statistical reports that create forums for complicated discussions. This statistical work eventually is distilled down to a conclusion. The paucity of proven interventions supports the need for an additional methodology, because statistical analysis will continue unabated even without any positive effects.

Many thousands of scientific papers reflect the billions of dollars and countless hours spent on sepsis research projects, but this extreme commitment has found no answers nor provided new medications or therapies.

Sepsis seems to be less a solitary disease and more of an aggressive destructive process that results in organ damage and/or death. Other diseases also present with clinical problems that are similar to those present in sepsis and must be rapidly differentiated for proper treatments to be applied.

The research descriptions provide precise elements and functions of physiologic systems, which are essential to support the development of a new disease pathway concept. These published studies preserve and amplify our knowledge of the unbelievable complexity of human physiology. However, much of the data found and concurrently reported does support the actions presented in this new concept of inflammation and cytokine storm.

The current focus is on specific chemical alterations that can be measured during the onset of sepsis. The chemical compounds released into the circulation at the onset of sepsis theoretically should provide identifiable patterns to facilitate the rapid diagnosis and differentiation of the sepsis process. Sadly, the chemical and data analyses still cannot (do not) tell when sepsis is happening. These research probes have been of little value for the prediction of the severity of the course or of the medical illness of patients with sepsis.

The recognition of an essential diagnostic algorithm to identify sepsis remains an elusive goal. The search for a solution goes on and on. But until an algorithm is defined and accepted, computer assisted diagnosis (artificial intelligence) cannot be accomplished.

Sepsis is still limited to clinical recognition, using fever, tachycardia, hyperpnea, decreased perfusion, and confusion as the sepsis markers. The clinician at the bedside must come to the correct diagnosis and quickly. Better outcomes are shown to happen with rapid diagnosis and immediate interventive treatments. The scientific work on identification and rapid response therapies continues unabated.

Today all critical care practitioners recognize sepsis with its varied manifestations of disease presentation. The medical practitioners accept these variances as customary when a diagnosis is needed.

Sepsis is presumed to be the response to an infectious stimulation by definition, but some other undefined stimulus, at least, mimics sepsis.

The inflammatory cytokine reaction is dramatic and huge in its natural presentation. The leukocyte response to infection has been compared to hunting rabbits with grenades; so much surrounding tissue damage results. "We have met the enemy and it is us!"

The pattern of human response varies widely. The group of interleukins causes fever and accelerated physiologic responses. Coagulation (clotting) occurs, and the thrombin system is activated. Circulatory instability and extracellular fluid loss presents as shock, also related to the cytokine storm.

Therapeutic response with fluid interventions often results in fluid overload of the organs. This has given rise to Multiorgan Dysfunction Syndrome (MODS) that progresses to organ failure and eventual death. The treatment routines are intensive, but the basic interventions modifying the pathophysiology remain quite minimal, and sadly do not alter the sepsis process very much.

Some patients will live and some patients will die, but the causes of the different courses the individual patients follow are still unknown and rarely even discussed in speculation about the dying process.

The current status of medical treatment does nothing to help! Once the status of "no cure available" is recognized, the medical response is fear and panic, this fear is magnified by the leaders responsible for the actual pandemic management. Too little data is available, and the medical experience needed for the interpretation is not present. This is an untenable situation.

Premature erroneous conclusions usually result in improper actions, but these interventions are supported by strong emotional commitments. These extraneous human emotional issues make the difficult situation even worse. The panic approach usually does not lead to a clear thought process, good outcomes rarely are achieved.

All the theories and interventions must be validated to avoid useless expensive treatments that end up helping no one.

Not only are pandemics difficult, but uncontrolled disease adds stress and fear to the community and the medical profession.

These are impossible situations that require many unsupported decisions. Each decision is made with the full knowledge that this decision alone may or may not be correct.

Change brings insecurity.

Louis Pasteur wrote, "The greatest derangement of the mind is to believe something because one wishes it to be true."

But the harsh reality is that **it makes little difference what we do when there is no cure!**

CHAPTER TWO

Tools We Do and Do Not Have to Treat Sepsis

Clinical Case: Another Early Critical Care Case

A seven-year-old girl was being transferred because of progressive breathing problems. She had a three-day history of cough, fever, and malaise. She failed to respond to antibiotics and bronchodilator treatments, and had become progressively worse quite rapidly.

Again, another emergency admission with the exact details submerged in the emotional context of her life and death. This story is another case presenting during the early phase of the Critical Care Medicine Specialty development. It clearly shows the dearth of knowledge in the early years of medical specialty development.

She, at age seven, was such a thin, frail child, but quite strong. She worked to do everything anyone asked her to do, even when it was difficult for her. She could only be described as a very sweet child.

She had not been sick for long, but her breathing problems seemed to just steadily get worse to the point she could do little to help herself.

Her treatments with oxygen, antibiotics, and bronchodilators were not effective, although they were medically classified as early interventions.

On admission, she was blue in color, with very rapid breathing. Neurologically, she was slow to respond to verbal stimuli and at times seemed to be delirious. Her vital signs showed a pulse of 180 beats per minute, blood pressure of 70/30, and perfusion was a slow return to her initial skin color. Just watching her was frightening, and everyone just knew she was critically ill and likely to die.

The immediate treatment was a rapid sequence intubation and full ventilatory support with 100 percent oxygen. She was monitored via an arterial line, which allowed measurement of blood pressure and blood gas measurements to assess the ventilation and adjust the ventilator.

Despite the full support, these interventions were unable to get arterial blood gas oxygen to normal and to get the CO^2 down to the normal range (which caused persistent respiratory failure). This "primitive ventilator" was difficult to manage; the desired settings provided were very simple.

Increasing the ventilator pressures resulted in the development of severe barotrauma with bilateral pneumothoraxes and interstitial air on the chest x-ray. These complications became progressively unmanageable problems. She developed refractory respiratory failure and died a classic sepsis death.

The treatment she was given was what seemed to be the best course of management during early Critical Care. So much has changed, all for the better.

The clinical course review showed the current interventions and the pattern of support provided was state of the art but, in retrospect, was inadequate. This child's case is so hard to even think about, and that limits discussion of the disease course. The only conclusion from the case review was that somewhere, somehow a treatment would be found.

Her death was an enduring force that continuously fed my sense of urgency to find a solution.

Building a sense of knowledge about sepsis is difficult. To start and to build an understanding of this immensely complicated disease and the medical environment, below is a review of some of the current medical treatment patterns.

Medicine is not too difficult to understand in small pieces, but the volume is huge and each individual item is described clearly and can be understood once the medical vocabulary is learned. The sheer volume of this seemingly foreign terminology overwhelms all the learners at the start. Success comes to those who work steadily and slowly to build their knowledge and understanding of "Medicine."

The limited discussion of standardized research provides a backdrop to build an awareness of the difficulties in medicine. Each change brings benefits to the medical treatments that endure today.

The clinical application of our sophisticated medical activities and treatments today are sadly only supportive measures. When the treatment plan for a medical condition is searched for and found in a major medical text, the likely textbook answer is to provide "supportive measures."

To the general population, this "answer" of supportive care is clearly deficient. The answers lack sufficient direction and provide minimal precision. Therefore, all medical plans seem unfocused and very vague.

To the early students of medicine, supportive measures are:

> These answers are inadequate. Too little and too brief to provide competent comprehensive direction for patient management.

To the young physician, supportive measures are:

> These answers are limited and largely unstructured, seemingly incomplete. Often the textbooks provide insufficient direction and limited specific direction.

To the experienced clinician, supportive measures are:

> The answer for supportive care is "more supportive care."

"Do more of the same old stuff" and "support each organ" as failure occurs with highly technical interventions to compensate for functional organ failure and functional loss.

Do the best that you can and as early as possible and then hang in there.

These answers are clearly problematic to all.

Medical supportive measures that are readily available today include:

- Intravenous fluids when oral intake is inadequate to maintain fluid balance and nutrition
- Antibiotics for infectious disease etiologies
- Antiviral drugs for viral infections
- Infusion of antibodies for specific disease states
- Administration of antifungal medication for fungal infections
- Administration of oxygen when oxygen levels are decreased.
- Pharmaceutical agents to control blood pressure (both high and low blood pressures), diuretics to increase urine flow, and other specific interventions as the conditions worsen
- Ventilator to be used when breathing function is mechanically impaired
- Extra Corporeal Membrane Oxygenator (ECMO) to support or replace lung and/or heart function
- Dialysis machine to replace kidney function
- Blood components to manage coagulation and anemia
- Drug Infusions to treat thrombosis and prevent complications
- Prophylactic antibiotics to prevent secondary infection
- Systemic steroids as a general supportive measure
- And all other interventions that could possibly be of some help must also be added

These unique clinical practice skills define the practice of the specialty of Critical Medicine. These supportive measures are very complex skills and require a great deal of knowledge and experienced judgment combined with technical mechanical skills in the application and use.

While treatment is limited, these medical interventions are truly supportive of the patients throughout their illnesses. Their appropriate application really does save many lives.

Even though these measures are only supportive and are not curative, they are very helpful. These interventions keep the patient alive with the hope the patient will live long enough to use his own body's healing measures to survive the disease.

Something new is needed to change or stop the disease progression.

When providing direct patient care, there is a desperate need for the clinician at the bedside to "do something more." But all too frequently, all the caregivers can only watch while the patient deteriorates and death approaches.

Are there any answers to these common questions?

Why do some people survive and yet others die?

No answer or even suggestions.

Why do some people die very rapidly, and other patients linger for long periods?

We do not know!

Why isn't being strong and healthy a guarantee of survival?

We still do not know!

How can some elderly weak individuals survive while others die of the same or very similar disease?

That answer would be helpful!

Herein Lies the Mystery of Life

How can someone strengthen their innate immune system?

> No answer: much is said, but nothing can be found that can be shown to work.

What is the role of individual genetic pattern in inflammatory diseases?

> Again, there has been extensive study but no answers. A huge amount of time and especially money is looking down this road for answers not yet found …

Is the genome going to find an answer?

> So far, looking via the genetic studies have found nothing helpful. But some clues keep the search going.

Why doesn't everyone have the same disease pattern with the same cause?

> Or maybe they all do?

These are the unanswered questions that apply to all scientists, caregivers, families, and patients alike. Certainly, countless other questions quickly come to mind to further our attempt to define the problems, but these additional probing questions still have no answers.

The responsibility of the physician and the medical team is to provide the best medical supportive care in the timeliest manner. While providing care, the physician must be absolutely certain that everything is precisely and correctly executed.

Yet despite exactly correct measures performed by the entire team, some of our patients still go on to die; too many, too soon, despite everyone's best efforts.

When a person/patient dies, this patient's death is a very personal and individual failure. All the members of the medical team, all of whom were responsible for the patient's care, feel this death very deeply and as a personal loss.

This is a good response, as positive and caring interactions develop during the support process. Denial is not an effective method of compensation.

These "unavoidable deaths" are all too frequent and are common to all in Critical Care. The social pressure continues to build a state of anxiety and fear in each caring caregiver as the deaths continue. Many recurrent episodes of patient demise eventually lead to stress-induced severe depression and Post Traumatic Stress Disorder (PSTD).

This over-stressed situation results in an unmanageable situation for any caring and treating team, which leads to a situation referred to as "burnout."

Physician burnout results from the unrelieved stress of Critical Care. This stress has become worse during Covid-19 pandemic. Burnout now extends to all levels of care providers and has become a major problem in health care at all levels.

The recognition and especially the realization of **"no cure for my patient"** is an exceedingly difficult truth to accept. Most caregivers do not or cannot accept this reality. This item is buried in denial.

This antithetical reality is especially difficult for the caring individual physicians and nurses to accept. This internal conflict builds to a tension-loaded situation.

Often, this tension leads to unsupported clinical controversies presented with great individual fervor, but still without answers. This stress of unmanageable progressive disease continues the strong demand for answers. The premise that anything is better than nothing now becomes an undesirable option for many. Individual conflicts and stress resulting from these unproven interventions and these allegations only make the situation worse. The basis of these conflicts is a true desire to help that cannot happen.

Today, data becomes the "answer." When conflicting evidence is presented, everyone has the opportunity to choose their own answer. Picking one viewpoint is easily available to them.

The medical community knows the limitations of their medical treatment, but the individual caregivers must continue to provide full support despite recognizing a poor prognosis for that patient. The need for continuing supportive care is clearly a very valuable service, even when all these actions are futile.

But the basic problem of **how to move** (treat sepsis) **the unmovable objec**t (sepsis) remains the constant problem today).

Frustration, combined with recognition of the futility of treatments and disease randomness, brings innate fear and breeds professional dysfunction.

The general population is aware of stress, but they, too, are afraid and are powerless to affect changes. Most people understand and appreciate the efforts and commitments of the physicians and caregivers without linkage to the outcome.

Everyone knows the tools in our possession to treat disease are inadequate. This treatment limitation problem is avoided and rarely discussed. Eventually, the question is answered by presenting a supporting a new plan of "continuing scientific research."

A pertinent summary of each medical life-changing episode can help everyone begin to understand the extremely difficult dynamics involved in the process of consistent and inconsistent changes that are a part of life survival patterns.

Our current scientific research approach is working to find a "cure" hidden somewhere in the huge amount of scientific information by "mining" this data using computer analysis. The future is included in this huge amount of data, or maybe it is someplace else. Maybe the computer can save us. Let us hope that artificial intelligence will help to find the answer, but that effort will need physician creativity.

Our individual human search programming must go on if change is ever to happen.

But the problem is:

Where should it go?

What to search for?

So much scientific information is available, but can that body of knowledge be sorted to provide direction to the scientific community? The answer is: Not yet.

A brief, focused, historical review of medical "miracles" or clinical breakthroughs will help to understand how change happens in medicine, as it has over the years.

This review of the medical science provided here is very superficial and brief. Hundreds of thousands of reports are available; a quantity far beyond anyone's capacity to know and understand.

This book is a small, focused attempt to provide enough scientific information to help build a further understanding of our problems and the ongoing research process. This book will eventually develop the foundation to bring a new theory of the disease process, and a product to intervene is presented here.

Once again, this presentation is focused on the gross changes experienced clinically rather than the exacting and minutely fine details of the most scientific experiments. Research is critical to the advancement of medicine, but too often in the practice of medicine action is needed before the whole conclusion is even understood.

Some answers are here in this discussion of a little-known human body organ with essential functions contained in a relatively new region of this "organ" of the body. This region is known as the endothelial glycocalyx—the glycocalyx (gli-co-cay-lix) and endothelial (en-do-the-li-al) cells.

This endothelial glycocalyx system (organ) is a relatively newly-appreciated and most important yet poorly understood essential organ system. This role of endothelial glycocalyx will be discussed in depth in a coming chapter, as this topic will require an additional information base to provide the basis for the new explanation of sepsis.

Within this new organ system contains the answer to more and better treatment of human illnesses.

All these changes in the understanding of the inflammatory cascade have been discovered by integrating our basic science research and the observations during the provision of complex critical care to our patients.

"In the field of observation, chance favors only the prepared mind." -Louis Pasteur

CHAPTER THREE

Changing the World by Changing the Response

These stories show the effects of individuals who changed their world, and these actions now save our lives.

The world of disease does change, both on its own and, more importantly, because of man's actions. These are but some of the changes brought about by dedicated individuals determined to find answers. The world today greatly underappreciates these men and women and their miracles that keep us alive today.

In 1979, the World Health Organization declared the entire world to be free of the disease **smallpox**. The entire world worked together to make this miracle happen. This too was a miracle, the whole world (all the people and the counties) working together to save all our lives. Such a difficult concept today, e.g., working for the good of all!

This is such a remarkable achievement started by treating the few and eventually becoming an accomplishment of huge magnitude. This smallpox eradication is so underappreciated today. Millions, or more likely billions of people have been saved by the simple process of vaccination.

Our medical care today is assumed by most people to "just be here" and expected to function with little or no thought.

How, what, and by whom did the medical care that benefits us all today happen?

The Covid-19 pandemic showed that problems still existed and there were no easy answers, and too few ready to search and find that answer.

"Those critical thinkers will just show up," they thought.

That is what has happened in the past.

There were six remarkable men throughout history who, with their creativity and persistent focus, changed the entire world of untreatable illnesses and problems. The following stories of miracles in medicine are only a few of the great numbers of medical discoveries that help us survive. Who will make similar changes to better our future?

History likes to attribute the great breakthroughs in medicine to a single defined individual physician working in isolation, but the reality is that many people were working in the same general area of medical science, and all were thinking and acting concurrently. These colleagues and even the competitors were a vital part of the active medical community and provided the knowledge backdrop that established the opportunity. This is the same medical community that initially provided resistance but would come to recognize, accept, adopt, and propagate these discoveries eventually. These changes and the adoption of new ways do not come easily at any time or place. Credit all our ancestors for the recognition and adoption of these new concepts.

This same medical community must go on to adopt and facilitate the application of the latest changes for the betterment of contemporary medical care.

There is a glacial progression of science through the ages, ever forward but slowly.

These accomplishments of our medical forefathers are almost inconceivable when the limited sophistication and the primitive status of their medical settings are considered. The severity of the problem that each individual recognized was of such importance that each individual maintained their focus and persevered to eventually carry out medical miracles.

The determination and the courage that was necessary for the individual physicians to make a change is so very hard to comprehend. The patterns of abuse within society were then and remain today such negative destructive forces.

A challenge to the status quo is so threatening and so disruptive that any action is hard to contemplate, and worse yet, worthy of destruction. Things are not better today.

Only six of medicine's greatest accomplishments are included in this chapter, and then only briefly in summary.

These stories of outstanding achievement are supplied to build an understanding of the surrounding situations that led to these revolutionary medical accomplishments.

The many other wonderful contributions to medicine have not been included. They have not been ignored, but only omitted because all these major contributions could not be included here.

These six stories were chosen as examples of the determination and perseverance needed to make the world change.

Hippocrates was the first, and truly revolutionized medical interactions forever. **Edward Jenner** eliminated a disease from the face of the earth. **Thomas Latta** brought patient/physician interaction into medical care. **Ignaz Semmelweis** recognized the spread of infection could be limited by handwashing. **Louis Pasteur,** while not a physician, was determined to make changes in medical practices and to have these changes be accepted. **Alexander Fleming** took a simple observation and pursued the development of penicillin for more than seventeen years to a successful end.

Hippocrates has been given the title of **Father of Medicine**.

Hippocrates transformed medical care with the transfer of direct medical care from the priests and the religious temples to the physicians. This action forced a change resulting in the abandonment of the code of established secrecy held by the priest control. The physicians were established to be the provider of medical care for all ill people.

Hippocrates brought the illnesses of mankind out into the open air through community forum discussions. The disease conditions were openly discussed. This transparency of open discussions established the principles of honesty and truthfulness. **These principles of honesty and truthfulness established the basis of medicine forever.**

Hippocrates developed or was credited with the Hippocratic Oath. That document established truth and honesty as the basic ethical components for the practice of medicine. The development of principles of treatments and the commitment to integrity of the physicians in medicine have been adopted and have survived centuries and should remain forever.

How much controversy and social upheaval in the Greek world this change caused can only be speculated. Undoubtedly, these new actions were disruptive action in Greek society of Hipporcrates time. Certainly, the Code of Hippocrates was adopted by all "physicians" of the time. The passage of these basic ethical rules has been passed on from physician to physician. These rules have become an essential basis of the profession of physician.

The priest healers gradually disappeared from mainstream medicine.

Today, we now have free and open discussions with the full expectations of total honesty in all forms of medical information.

The Hippocratic Oath that instilled integrity into the physicians is the eternal contribution of Hippocrates. This oath alone would be adequate to secure his recognition as the Father of Medicine.

Edward Jenner (d. 1823) is credited with the development of a vaccine to prevent smallpox. He used and modified the techniques then known in his time.

Smallpox was the major scourge of mankind for millennia, causing death to about a third of the world's population. Deaths due to smallpox were even identified in Egyptian mummies. This disease caused recurrent epidemics and altered the histories of all the great powers of the world.

The populations and the dynamics of the political world were altered by huge epidemics of smallpox.

Smallpox epidemics were spread by conquering armies and affected the outcomes of wars from Europe to Japan. The plague of Athens in 450 BCE, the Antonine Plague in the Roman Empire in 165-180 AD, and the Japanese epidemic of 733-737 AD—each killed a third of the populations. Epidemics throughout the world created immeasurable disruption and population rearrangements in every continent.

Smallpox was the worst infectious disease ever known to affect mankind.

A practice named variolation apparently originated in China in the fifteenth century using the pus exudate material from the lesions of smallpox disease. This pus was inoculated into the skin of patients using various methods to break the skin integrity. This treatment (variolation) caused only a mild disease condition, usually, but provided lifetime protection against smallpox.

This procedure became known but only slowly spread across the world and was applied primarily in the aristocracy. There was mortality when too much Inoculum was used, and the failed attempt to prevent smallpox actually caused active severe smallpox disease and led to death in those cases. This complication of variolation created uncertainty and limited widespread variolation adoption.

Edward Jenner was variolated as a child and therefore had lifetime immunity to smallpox.

Jenner was trained as a physician in England. He apprenticed with John Hunter, a physician, who when traditional medical methods failed was reputed to try new, different methods. Jenner learned medicine and science from Dr. Hunter and was also trained to search for answers. He was open-minded, and therefore able to review and analyze the smallpox disease problem.

Jenner worked to define smallpox and cowpox, but the scientific means could not clearly differentiate the "poxes" from each other.

Jenner became aware of the association between cowpox and smallpox. He noted that the two pox diseases had very different courses in people. He noted that the milkmaids who had cowpox infections had immunity to smallpox disease. He combined this observation with his known understanding of the variolation procedure.

He further defined in his observations that the cowpox disease (pus) had to be at maximum strength (eighth day of disease) to be an effective vaccine inoculum (adequate amount of viral inoculum present at that time of the cowpox disease).

The first vaccination occurred on May 14, 1796. Jenner applied cowpox pus from Sarah Nelmes to variolation scratches on James Phipps. Jenner later repeated the variolation procedure with smallpox disease pus to James Phipps, but this procedure did not cause any reaction, especially smallpox.

James Phipps became the first person ever to be immune to the smallpox disease after cowpox vaccination.

In 1778, a smallpox outbreak occurred. All those persons inoculated with cowpox were spared from the disease; a remarkably successful result.

Edward Jenner recorded his findings and attempted to publish this information. The Royal Society of Medicine refused to publish his findings, citing a "lack of evidence."

Dr. Jenner then rode to London, where he wrote and published his book, *An Inquiry into the Causes and Effects of the Variola Vaccinaea* in 1798.

This book established the vaccination procedure. Vaccination was then accepted throughout the medical world, but the spread of vaccination was slow in its application.

The limiting factor was that cowpox was an uncommon disease. Virus (yet unknown) for the inoculum made only a very small amount of cowpox virus pus during its infection, so the vaccine supply from cowpox was very scarce and difficult to obtain. This limited the number of vaccinations.

The modern methods of viral culture ultimately eliminated this obstruction to vaccine production and widespread application of vaccinations immediately followed.

Across the world, the vaccination programs for smallpox were extremely effective. Smallpox as a disease was eradicated in 1979 by the World Health Organization's mass vaccination effort. **This is the first human disease totally eradicated by vaccination**. This is a scientific medical miracle. Dr Edward Jenner's work has probably saved more lives through his vaccine development than any other medical advancement ever. It also was a worldwide political miracle!

Thomas Latta (d. 1833) in 1834 reported in the *Journal Lancet* the first use ever of intravenous fluids to resuscitate a patient. This was during a severe cholera outbreak in 1832 in Edinburgh, Scotland.

Dr. Latta had worked with **Sir William Brooke O'Shaughnessy,** who determined the blood of severely ill patients was deficient in water, salt, and free alkali. O'Shaughnessy made the suggestion that replenishing salts would lead to patient recovery. He did not ever apply that knowledge.

Dr. Thomas Latta's report of this first intravenous intervention administering fluids is so dramatic that it had to be included as originally presented.

This report is from the *Edinburgh Medical Journal* (37), 1832.

Imagine the primitive hospital setting that existed in 1830. Imagine the emotional setting, knowing with certainty of the imminent death of the patient.

Then, follow along with this letter by Dr Latta to the Central Board of Health in Edinburg:

> I attempted to restore the blood to its natural state by injecting copiously into the larger intestines warm water. Trusting that the power of absorption might not all together be lost, but by these means I produced, in no case any permanent benefit. I at length, resolved to throw the fluid immediately into the circulation. In this, having no precedent to direct me, I proceeded with much caution. The first subject was an aged female. She had apparently reached the last moments of her Earthly existence and now nothing could injure her—indeed, so entirely was she reduced that I feared I should be unable to get my apparatus ready ere she expired. Having inserted a tube into the Basilic Vein, cautiously anxiously, I watched the effects; ounce after ounce was injected. But no visible change was produced. Still persevering, I thought she began to breathe less laboriously, soon the sharpened feature and the sunken eye and fallen jaw pale and cold bearing the manifest impress of death's signet, began to glow with returning animation; the pulse which had long ceased, returned to the wrist; at first small and quick, by degrees it became more and more distinct….and in the short space of half an hour, and when six pints had been injected, she expressed in a firm voice that she was free of all uneasiness, actually became jocular, and fancied all she needed was a little sleep.

This report of the results was published in *The Lancet* on June 23, 1832.

This *Lancet* article graphically illustrates the treatment:

> The very remarkable effects of the remedy require to be witnessed to be believed. Shortly after the commencement of the injection the pulse, which was not perceptible, gradually returns; the eyes, which were sunk and turned upwards, are

suddenly brought forward, and the patient looks round as if in health, the natural heat of the body is gradually restored, the tongue and breath, which were in some cases at the temperature of 79° and 80°, rise to 88° and 90°, and soon become natural, the laborious respiration and oppression of weight of the chest are relieved . . . the whole countenance assumes a natural healthy appearance"[10]

This fluid that was specified by Dr. William Brooke O'Shaughnessy and used by Dr. Thomas Latta was difficult to make and exceeded the resources and the equipment capacity of the day. Therefore, inconsistent chemical solutions were produced, although the initial acceptance was generally positive about the benefit of fluids as lifesaving therapy; the procedure could not become therapy until the difficult problems of accurate measurements of sodium, potassium, bicarbonate, and chloride were later solved.

Thomas Aitchison Latta died in 1833 of tuberculosis.

Despite the multiple medical publications of the miracle fluid resuscitation, the practice of intravenous infusion was not continued to be performed. For the next seventy years, intravenous treatments were not performed.

Not until the year 1902 was intravenous therapy reintroduced as medical therapy. This therapy was still very slowly adopted into medical therapy, specifically due to many technical problems with equipment and the limited availability of the correct fluids to be given.

Today, treatment with intravenous fluids is routine. Far too few people know of the courageous contribution of Thomas Latta.

Ignaz Semmelweis, born July 1, 1818, died August 13, 1865, is recognized as the pioneer of antiseptic procedures.

Dr. Semmelweis observed childbirth fever was much less frequent with women who had "street births" than births in the Hungarian birthing centers.

He linked the death of a colleague who received an incidental stab wound during an autopsy, and subsequently died of a condition that was similar to that of the many women who were dying of puerperal fever (childbirth fever).

Semmelweis then concluded the instruments carried "cadaverous materials" that caused his associate's death. This concept of "cadaveric contamination" became the basis of his chlorine solution for hand washing.

Semmelweis used a chlorine solution because it also eliminated the stench from the cadavers, and incidentally also destroyed the causal poisonous agents.

The simple observation resulted in a change in procedure, and practitioners began the use of hand washing with a chlorine solution.

This single change to hand washing resulted in a huge decrease in puerperal fever deaths by 90 percent. The rate decreased from 18.3 percent to 2.2 percent in two months. In one year, there were no deaths for the same two-month period.

Despite the well-documented report using an easily measured parameter, community acceptance was at best grudging. Controversy was the best description.

The reason for the lack of endorsement that is currently receiving the most credence is **"belief perseverance"** of this pathbreaking contribution. This is referred to as the **Semmelweis Reflex,** which is the resistance to change and "constitutes the most formidable block to scientific advances."

Some physicians were offended because their social status as gentleman was incompatible with unclean hands that could be the cause of death.

Political turmoil of the time included multiple revolutions in many European countries. The Hungarian Revolution of 1848 occurred simultaneously with the discoveries by Dr. Semmelweis. Whether these general political changes or the more subtle local politics were the dominant causes of the controversies is unclear.

The initial reports were published by his colleagues who, at times, were unclear in their descriptions. He reported that he left Vienna because he was "unable to endure further frustration in dealing with the Vienna medical establishment." His medical career did not flourish.

Clearly, his professional relationships were not positive. He became angry and lashed out at his critics and colleagues. He called them names, including "murderers and ignoramuses." His outbursts were "highly polemical and superficially offensive."

His writings were demeaned, and he became progressively antagonistic and overtly angry. He eventually turned to alcohol and developed behavioral aberrancies for which he was hospitalized in a mental institute. Whether this deterioration was due to syphilis (an inherent disease risk factor for obstetricians of that era) or something else, we shall never know.

In this mental facility, he was beaten and sustained an injury to his hand. His hand became severely infected. Ironically, Dr. Semmelweis died of sepsis.

This historical review clearly shows these years were not a proud time in medical development. The discovery was monumental, but almost all physicians of note derided and ridiculed this monumental breakthrough.

An additional long-lasting result of his tumultuous life is the very negative **"Semmelweis Reflex"** behavior, which is "behavior characterized by reflex-like rejection of new knowledge because it contradicts entrenched norms, beliefs, or paradigms."

Just imagine how infuriating the responses were in 1861, but even today these intense negative attitudes persist all too widely.

Ignaz Semmelweis at the time of his death received little recognition. Time has judged him to be a "Physician of Great Impact," recognizing the importance of hand washing (hygiene) in the treatment of what is now defined as sepsis.

A statue honoring Inaz Semmelweis stands in front of Szent Rokus Hospital in Budapest in recognition of his contribution to all mankind. Semmelweis University of Medicine, Semmelweis Klinik, and two hospitals named Semmelweis honor him in his native country.

His contribution is one that has never been adequately appreciated. Hand washing now seems such a simple, logical thing to do.

Louis Pasteur, born December 27, 1822, and died September 28, 1895.

He was a chemist and microbiologist. He was not a physician and had no medical training, but always worked within the medical institutions and was always at the forefront of the science era.

His long career covered a wide variety of issues during a time when ego and arrogance played a large role in the recognition of accomplishments.

His persistence is remarkable. **"Let me tell you the secret that has led me to my goal, my secret lies solely in my tenacity,"** he remarked.

Certainly, in the contentious world of medical science of the time in which he lived and worked, tenacity was a necessity. His quoted statements were undoubtedly used in some of the "discussions" in the halls of the science of that day.

"The greatest derangement of the mind is to believe in something because one wishes it to be true." This widely quoted statement was certainly used to "disembowel" the opposing debater. Still today, this contentious advocacy persists widely.

"The cold winters of Wisconsin have frozen your brain," a comment heard today, is a far less elegant insult to the opponent's presentations in his time. Extreme competition bred rudeness to colleagues. That incivility still exists today. The scientific world can be harsh.

Pasteur's accomplishments benefit everyone every day. The

procedure of "pasteurization" is so much an integral aspect of our food chain and other aspects of our essential product safety. The prevention of transmission of infections and the preservation of countless products for consumption is a result of his scientific study.

Pasteur recognized bacteria and its relationship to disease and supplied documentation for all to see.

Pasteur eliminated all discussion of spontaneous generation of life (bacteria). The problem of contamination was poorly appreciated.

Pasteur showed that when broth was boiled and placed in a container that did not allow air contamination, no growth occurred, but when air was allowed to enter the container, fermentation did occur. The presence of bacteria on the dust in the air contaminated the broths used in the studies, allowing growth. **No spontaneous generation! End of sentence concluded!**

Rabies was a deadly disease, and Pasteur's work on rabies is legendary. He developed a vaccine to treat those affected with rabies and was determined to treat victims of the disease. Pasteur was not a physician, and therefore had to accept the risk of legal prosecution when he treated a child with rabies. Fortunately, the patient survived and the potential prosecution for the practice of medicine without a license was not pursued. Nothing was easy or safe at that time.

At the time, a test for the rabies virus was not available. The rabies treatments still to this day are attributed to the work of Louis Pasteur.

Pasteur's contributions are many, but only after attracting controversy initially. After a century, his contributions are accepted and appreciated. The principles he developed have withstood the test of time.

Pasteur's legacy includes the multiple Pasteur Institutions across the world that are active in the support of human health activities.

Upon review of all he had accomplished, His statement "Let me tell you the secret that has led me to my goal, **MY STRENGHTH LIES SOLEY IN MY TENACITY**" summarizes how he did it all.

He is owed so much by everyone.

Alexander Fleming, born August 6, 1881 and died March 11, 1955.

He was trained as a physician, but he also worked in research on bacteria, and **he discovered penicillin.**

Major discoveries are not simple today, and this was in our modern world. No accomplishments are associated without extraordinary determination and commitment. Dr. Fleming had those admirable traits.

Dr. Fleming was a well-trained and well-respected British physician. During a tour of duty in World War I, he noted and reported antiseptics did not kill the bacteria in the deep wounds; these were largely gram-negative bacteria. Those soldiers with deep wounds infected with gram-negative bacteria often fared worse. As usual, this medical information was disquieting and was ignored and disparaged (this is the Semmelweis reflex manifested).

After the war he returned to his position as professor of bacteriology at St. Mary's Hospital in London. In the course of his work, he noted a lytic area on a petri dish around a piece of his own mucus. He found that product in many tissues and named it lysozyme.

The lecture "On a remarkable bacteriolytic element found in tissues and secretions" was received politely but created little if any interest. He invested a large amount of work in this discovery and carefully catalogued and defined all aspects of this lysozyme entity.

Fleming's work on lysozymes was recognized and earned him a reputation as a brilliant researcher.

The discovery of penicillin is a legendary story deservedly retold and retold.

Fleming himself comments on the discovery and these comments reveal a lot about his life and character: "One sometimes finds what one is not looking for. *When I woke up just after dawn on September 28, 1928, I certainly did not plan to revolutionize all medicine by discovering the world's first antibiotic, or bacteria killer. But I suppose that was exactly what I did."*

This shows what type of a man he truly was.

This first story is an edited and simplified version of the story of penicillin discovery story.

Dr. Fleming, following his established pattern of leaving the laboratory menial scut work incomplete, left on a vacation without fully cleaning up his laboratory work area. How much is legend and how much is reality just makes the story better.

In another and more accurate story, Dr. Fleming inoculated culture plates with staphylococcus. On his return from vacation, he noted that amongst his culture plates (petri dishes), one had been contaminated with a fungus and the area around the fungus had a clear "kill zone" where the staphylococci should have grown. On the periphery the staphylococci were normal.

Dr. Fleming immediately recognized this unusual condition and knowingly pursued this discovery. The fungus eventually identified as penicillium had produced something that killed the staphylococcus.

Dr. Fleming presented, wrote, and published these findings on this new bacterial-killing phenomenon. Few other researchers understood and appreciated the true value of this discovery.

Dr. Fleming continued his work in his laboratory to better define the characteristics of **penicillin**.

The research product was named after the fungus that elaborated the killing essence, penicillium. Hence the name **penicillin**.

The research was difficult and testing was compromised by the difficulty of obtaining adequate amounts of penicillin. The chemists working on the penicillin project actually declared the isolation and chemical purification of penicillin to be a futile exercise. But still the work continued under the supervision of Dr. Fleming.

The ensuing years were the forgotten years of Fleming and penicillin. During the 1936 Second International Congress of Microbiology, which was held in London, Dr. Fleming's presentation of the penicillin discovery generated little to no interest in the disease treatment possibilities. The Congress concluded that penicillin was a product with little value.

In 1942, an article in the *British Medical Journal* reported, "Penicillin does not appear to have been considered as a possibly useful product from any other point of view."

The years following the world's greatest discovery, followed by a minimal recognition of this breakthrough discovery, were very difficult and disappointing.

Dr. Fleming undertook a very complicated and difficult search for new manufacturing technique. The steps that were needed to make large amounts of penicillin almost cost the world this wonderful discovery. The years without success resulted in his "abandoning" penicillin development.

This myth of Fleming is not true. His role and interest in penicillin never waned. Despite the total lack of support, Fleming continued to work developing penicillin.

Dr. Fleming left the final phase of actual production development to his colleagues, with instructions to "finish the job." However, Fleming continued to be involved in penicillin development.

At the Radcliff infirmary at Oxford, the team of Ernst Boris Chain and Howard Florey took up the research to mass-produce penicillin. The funding was provided by the U.S. and British governments to fund crisis developments to support World War II projects. The dates for funding are vague. After the team at Oxford published the positive results in 1940, Dr. Fleming called Earnst Boris Chain to announce he was coming to visit Oxford, to which Dr. Chain allegedly responded, "Good God! I thought he was dead."

Norman Heatley assisted in the modification of the essential manufacturing techniques that allowed mass production of penicillin. Readily available quantities were needed to provide sufficient amounts of penicillin for clinical trials.

The molecular structure of penicillin was defined by Edward Abraham, who characterized the correct structure of the penicillin molecule.

With the whole team at Oxford working on penicillin development as a war effort, a stable product form was rapidly developed. Animal trials were able to be performed and clinical studies could be completed.

Subsequently, the team developed the methods of mass production and mass distribution. This emergency penicillin war effort was so successful that by D-Day in 1944, enough penicillin was available to treat all the Allied troops.

After the war in 1945, enough penicillin was produced to begin to treat all who needed penicillin therapy.

This post-World War II period began the modern era of antibiotics in medicine.

Alexander Fleming did live to be recognized for his achievement as **the discoverer of penicillin.**

Alexander Fleming, Howard Florey, and Ernst Boris Chain were awarded the Nobel Prize for Medicine in 1945. These men are credited for the new era of antibiotic therapy in medicine.

These remarkable stories of difficulty and the responses from society, which varied from lack of appreciation to open direct abuse, are now difficult to believe.

These remarkable people persevered with strong personal beliefs and commitment to their science. Each one did eventually have their contributions recognized as an important step in the betterment of our human existence.

There were many other concurrent accomplishments, and there will be many more accomplishments to come.

These advancements in medical care required total courage of convictions and unbelievable persistence. When we contemplate these stories and the ramifications of these simple miracles, a sense of gratitude and appreciation is generated.

These gifts to all humankind did not come about easily. We honor these men today.

CHAPTER FOUR

Sepsis Treatments Today

Things are better but still the answer is not here.

The tertiary hospital accepts all transfers!

This disaster focuses on a 19-year-old male who had been connecting a hose from an anhydrous ammonia truck to a farm storage tank when something went wrong, and the pressurized anhydrous ammonia filled the whole area with this extremely toxic gas.

Details of his rescue were not clearly provided. Who found him, what was done, and how long it took to get help were never known.

He did have very severe inhalation damage to his lungs in addition to facial chemical burns and severe conjunctivitis. His upper airway and nasal passages were red and swollen.

He was intubated at the scene and brought to and assessed in the Emergency Department of an outlying hospital. An immediate transfer directly to the Pediatric Intensive Care Unit was made.

He required full ventilator support with high-end expiratory pressure and volume-controlled ventilation (the best technology of the day). Oxygen was administered at 100 percent and decreased as the blood gas levels allowed. His pulmonary status seemed to be manageable on this aggressive support. His electrolytes and pH levels were unusual as there was a metabolic alkalosis present, which was treated and did not recur. Renal function continued to be adequate with repeated fluid boluses and the urine output was acceptable.

Because of the extensive skin and mucus membrane damage and the need for respiratory control, both sedation and muscle relaxants (neuromuscular blockers) were used. Analgesics for pain control were continuously provided.

His hospital course was very difficult. The monitoring needed to integrate pulmonary function, urinary output, blood pressure, and electrolyte changes required constant attention. This was difficult but manageable. Wound care added to his care load.

Ammonium nitrate inhalation injury usually is such a severe injury that the patients invariably die very rapidly. This resulted in a very limited prior experience. The development of our treatment program was directly in response to his altered pathophysiology. However, this patient seemed to stabilize slowly on our program of judicious comprehensive support. The four days of stability and slow improvement made everyone hopeful for his recovery. "They call them patients, so we wait for them to recover."

Our medical support plan was that of expectant waiting. The fluid boluses caused generalized swelling of the entire body—everything, the worst being in his face. The mucus membranes were reddened and bulging, causing a very unpleasant swollen face with a barely identifiable nose. The swollen eyelids and red bulging conjunctival membranes were grossly disfigured. The leaking crusted plasma of the burn-like injuries and the dressings applied made a scene few ever before had seen. His body was very swollen as a result of the fluids and multiple transfusions that were required to support satisfactory circulation and blood pressure.

Still, all the organ systems seemed to be working. Maybe against all odds, we thought he could make it. The systems that could be supported seemed to be stable and improving.

On the fifth day, the plan to lighten the sedation and stop the paralysis (a sedation vacation) was instituted. When the neuromuscular blockers were stopped and the sedation eliminated, he had no response, he failed to awaken, and he had no neurological response at all.

What a devastating discovery! Everything had been done well and still, he died! Further neurologic testing confirmed the diagnosis of brain death.

Somewhere in this complex care milieu, his brain had died. No one knew when or how, or anything else!

His death was officially registered as a hypoxic insult and attributed to the ammonium inhalation gas injury that happened before effective interventions by the EMS at the scene.

What other process or other component of sepsis was working here?

This case was such a disappointment to all of us on the team. All the known parameters had been well managed, but still, he died.

The answer still evades us all. This post-care patient conference was a story of uncertainty and confusion. All the manageable parameters had been controlled adequately and promptly. What did we not know? What happened and when? Nobody had any answers or even productive thoughts.

The only answer was to keep watching and thinking and analyzing the information and caring for the people. Something would be found. Somehow.

Keep fighting the good fight!

Today, the general assumption of our society is **all is well in medicine.** Our medical system has the resources to cope with anything and everything that comes along. So be happy! Live with the myth.

However, the Covid-19 pandemic has clearly shown the limitations of our medical care today. When the disease strikes in its full force with sepsis, death certainly results. The limits of the supportive pattern of our complex medical care are painfully evident.

How and why some patients who are severely affected do survive is not known. Explanations are created and discussed. Many of these fervently-believed statements do not have the validity of anything other than sheer speculation. Certainly, our initial responses provided little to build upon.

What is the focus on the disease process that is addressed by today's scientific research? How and what is our point of attack? The analysis shows a surprising pattern of our limited interventions rarely if ever considered.

The entire focus is to end (kill) the pathogen! **Our singular solution to infectious disease is "Destroy the inciting cause before the disease begins."**

All the initial treatment modalities are metabolic interventions addressed to the physiology of the pathogen and are designed to disrupt the pathogen's function while not affecting the patient's physiology. Keep it away, and do not let it bother me!

Supporting, limiting, or **preventing the patient's inflammatory response** is not even an option. Though much is discussed, the reality is that there is nothing now in the medical armamentarium that can intervene to help the body stop the disease.

The entire mechanism of the existing interventions is to prevent disease development and is focused on killing the infecting organism and totally sparing the patient. The goal of medication is designed to avoid interfering with the metabolism of the affected patient.

All the therapies are designed to avoid placing any added stress on the body of the patient. There is nothing available for the host-patient physiologic reinforcement. There is nothing to help your patient out.

What then is available for the prevention and control of disease?

Isolation is the simplest and best preventive measure. No exposure; no disease.

Once an infectious agent is recognized within the community, the social planning for isolation use is considered and implemented. Mandated restriction to home. No visitors!

However, in our complex interconnected world, isolation is extremely difficult to carry out and in reality, is at best incomplete, even when conscientiously applied. And people have difficulty complying.

Hand washing is the first line of active defense. Hygiene; just plain old soap and water!

Sterilization technique is the most intensive phase of hygiene. Sterilization procedures are very effective at killing the bacteria and preventing bacterial access to humans. The pathogens are destroyed, and therefore eliminated prior to entering the patient. These items have all infecting agents on or within destroyed. Our tools are clean.

Vaccination is a preventive option. But **vaccination must be performed long before** the disease is present in the individual. The vaccine will cause a disease-like state that the immune system defines to develop specific immune responses only to that disease vaccine. With the next disease exposure, those antibodies will keep that specific infection from invading the patient. The pathogen is identified and destroyed before **the disease state begins. Vaccination works** whether the pathogen is viral, bacterial, or another agent **if done before the infection happens.**

Vaccination is a controlled infection like the specific condition but is mild. This product teaches the host (patient) about the infecting agent and allows it to create its own immune response. The current pattern of vaccine success is usually (historically) so good that the pathogen barely gets started before it is destroyed. And our greatest achievement using the tool of vaccination is the total eradication of smallpox from our entire world.

This is our best preventive medical treatment for almost all persons, but vaccination is not of benefit after an illness has begun. **Vaccination is specific for each infecting agent.**

Prior planning pays! **Get vaccinated for all preventable diseases.**

Antibodies are produced by the vaccinated or infected person and are found in the blood. Medical science has followed the vaccination response and has identified the antibody response. These beneficial components of the vaccination program are the products produced after the disease that prevent disease recurrence. The antibodies can be separated out and concentrated for use when that disease is starting to affect that patient.

These antibodies, specific for a single disease, start the immune response to prevent disease when transfused into a vulnerable exposed person. Antibody infusion prevents only the specific disease the antibodies were made to eliminate.

In the disease process, even when the inciting agent (bacteria) is killed or controlled, **the patient still must fix their own body.** Now starts the normal physiologic metabolic process of healing. If the inflammatory cascade has begun, the inflammatory response must be controlled and the damage caused by the inflammatory reaction must be healed. Certainly, nothing new. Food and supportive care for anyone who becomes infected is our maximum support.

Medical care today is a very sophisticated system of complex **supportive measures** combined with sophisticated knowledge of those supportive treatments.

Desperation weighs very heavily upon the caregivers, and that sense of desperation is made even more intense by the lack of any effective intervention to treat the underlying disease process.

In desperate times, the admonishment "physician do no harm" is essential and needs to be followed, especially in the situation when the supportive measures are not working. This is the time of desperation in each caregiver's life and can expose the patient to unproven risky treatments when futile efforts are being made.

The caregivers must accept the limitations of their ability to help each patient, but also accept the sad reality that the means to control the situation are sometimes not available to them.

The assurance that all known support has been applied appropriately and caringly allows the caregivers to continue their lifesaving efforts to provide the very best care.

The top administrators who can make decisions with minimal information and administer at a rapid pace, making rules and directives when there is a void in continuous medical decision-making, quickly move to take charge. Hence, some therapeutic programming lacks a sufficient basis for the actions proscribed.

Medically, sepsis causes body organ dysfunction and failure. Many of these metabolic needs can be handled with the replacement of the lost function for short periods of time. Sepsis causes physiologic failure of so many different organ functions and requires so much attention and interventional support. There are actions available for patient support of whatever disease is causing the body function failure. This interventional support means bringing technical medical items for specific functional support and substitution for lost function.

Almost all the essential physiologic and metabolic components that are limited or missing due to organ dysfunction can be provided. This deficiency ranges from totally absent to not enough made by the patient's failing organ. Almost all cases of organ failure can be supportively palliated. These products are administered to the patient for a limited time. Component replacement is a medical support treatment now frequently provided without much difficulty.

The supportive interventions are nearly unbelievable in their comprehensive interventions. These supports include the entire range of blood components and immunoglobulins and include administering fluids as needed, along with medications to support cardiac function and blood pressure. Adequate nutrition is necessary and when enteral feedings are inadequate; parenteral hyperalimentation provides the proteins, glucose, and fats along with vitamins and trace metals to compensate for enteral failure and more unlisted items.

Maintenance of near normothermia and avoidance of new compounding problems from the interventions are very essential basic support measures.

General hygiene along with nursing care must be maintained for each patient. These activities are very much underappreciated but essential. Prone positioning has been shown to benefit patients with severe pulmonary compromise. Techniques to prevent deep vein thrombosis are essential. Repositioning to avoid the development of pressure injuries is critical in this subset of patients with marginal cardiac output.

Circulatory volume support is provided via transfusion of blood products and crystalloid solutions. These infusions must be calculated to provide adequate intravascular volume. These products are usually required to be administered in huge volumes and carry the problem of third spacing and development of edema.

The current intensive care therapy fluid administration pattern is both lifesaving and potentially destructive.

The current fluid therapy is constantly being modified because the basic fluid leak (third spacing) problem is not yet solved. This aggressive fluid intervention has saved countless lives but cannot save them all. When fluids do not work and third spacing results, progression to death occurs via Multiorgan Dysfunction Syndrome (MODS).

The work on this fluid management is a continuing investigational program. This third spacing complication remains a major point of the pathophysiology of the sepsis syndrome.

MODS is the disease of current intensive care therapy. This syndrome is largely attributed to fluid management techniques, but also is a primary component of sepsis syndrome. The search for options and effective modifications of fluids continues with limited success.

Mechanical fluid removal is by ultrafiltration and dialysis help with fluid overload problems, but do not alter the disease progression.

Antibiotics are started as early as possible to prevent bacterial invasion. Antibiotic therapy is frequently added and continued or changed to prevent secondary bacterial infections.

Positive blood cultures are present in only one or two of three patients, and often no definitive site of etiology is found. In the few true cases of bacterial sepsis, the benefit of antibiotic use is to kill the inciting bacteria, and the earlier the better. The value of prolonged or continued antibiotic use can be argued (this is the basis for the sepsis protocols). Once the bacteria are killed there is no further benefit of antibiotic therapy.

Anti-fungal medications are usually reserved until a documented fungal infection is present. But for extremely high risk immunocompromised patients, anti-fungal treatments are sometimes added.

Antiviral medications are best used at illness onset or early in the disease. Late application has no benefit. These interventions are limited to the early period of infection to block or limit intracellular viral replication to perpetuate the infection. These antiviral medications stop viral reproduction only. But antiviral medications have no effect on the sepsis syndrome at any point.

The sepsis cascade is likely caused by more etiologies than infection. Only about 40 percent of the patients have initial positive blood cultures. The cytokine response occurs at the initiation of the inflammatory response. But because an inflammatory response occurs, antibiotics are customarily started early in most cases. You can't go back and do it; the "cytokine storm" may follow, and the sepsis syndrome progresses.

As the bodily functions fails, mechanical means are routinely applied.

Renal function is often impaired, and various forms of dialysis may be applied to manage this parameter. Mechanical dialysis against a specific solution can be used to correct abnormal electrolyte patterns and uremia often present. The dialysis technique returns the body to a normal or near-normal physiologic biochemical status. At times, ultrafiltration (removal of excess water) is used to adjust fluid volumes. No cure is provided at any point by using mechanical support for kidney failure.

Respiratory failure is treated by the application of a mechanical ventilator into the respiratory circuit. This machine does not treat disease; the ventilator just addresses mechanical ventilatory failure.

It does not increase the passage of oxygen from the alveolus to the capillary circulation. Ventilators only move air in and out of the lungs. When the muscles of respiration become fatigued and are too weak to supply the needed ventilation (air exchange) to meet the oxygenation and carbon dioxide requirements, mechanical assistance is provided.

However, the use of airway pressure itself creates stress damage to the lung tissue (called barotrauma). Even giving 100 percent oxygen creates damage patterns to the lung parenchyma. Respirator management is today an area that seems to be ideal for artificial intelligence management, but ventilator management still remains a clinical art form.

Nothing specifically stops acute respiratory distress syndrome (ARDS). When the ventilator using high pressures and 100 percent oxygen can no longer supply adequate oxygenation to the tissues, something more must be done immediately if the patient is to have any chance of survival.

The answer to lung failure is a complex medical support technique of Extra Corporeal Membrane Oxygenation (ECMO). This is where the blood is circulated through a machine with pumps attached to the arterial and venous connections to pump the blood across a specifically designed membrane that allows diffusion of oxygen into the blood and carbon dioxide (CO_2) to be diffused out of the blood. This circuit creates the required blood flow and removes CO_2 and delivers O_2. ECMO consumes so many valuable limited medical resources that the ECMO technique has limited availability for emergency patient rescue application.

The ultimate treatment of respiratory failure is a lung transplant (get a new lung). This is an extraordinarily expensive, complex process available to very few patients. The medical decision process to decide who can qualify for a lung transplant is one of the most difficult decisions in medicine today.

The pretransplant assessment includes:

1. A requirement that the patient must be expected to survive the lung transplant procedure.

2. Anticipation that the patient will have a long-term survival.

3. The transplant requires a donor whose death is unrelated to any process that causes damage to the lung.

Organ donorship is an exceedingly rare situation. It is certainly not a good answer to this nearly impossible situation; very few organs are available and then mostly from patients who have died.

Heart failure is one organ that is listed in the MODS list. Medications are the first line of interventions. Beyond that, the ECMO can also support circulatory failure by using pumps to drive blood circulation and blood pressure. The cannulas (tubes) are placed into the venous and arterial circulation to bypass the heart. ECMO is used for only a brief period of time in most cases.

Again, ECMO is a limited access procedure. The artificial heart usually is combined with ECMO programming. A large number of medical personnel and the general medical resources consumed through its use severely restrict the availability. Artificial heart technology is becoming more available, but it is still rare due to the huge quantity of resources needed for application. The limited number of medical centers that possess the capacity to provide and manage the artificial heart pump are few. Research into an artificial heart machine or simple pump is a reality today, but possible only in research institutions.

Heart transplants, while a possibility, are not an acute phase intervention and at present are not a part of the support for the septic patient.

Nutrition, fluid management, secondary prevention of infectious disease, replacement of blood, and other essential products are standard supportive measures. These basics often get pushed out by extremely complex interventions.

Disease treatment is a remarkably costly burden in all societies. No country has unlimited medical resources to be able to supply all means of medical support to all its citizens. The commitment to focus on all resources is common to every country. But even the USA cannot make all these interventions available to everyone.

Each government system across the globe decides and provides its own level of maximum support to its own population. However, reality speaks loud and clear. This is all there is today; these supportive measures are all that can be done.

These medical applications are complete and appropriate for the treatment of disease. An article in the June 2022 issue of *Critical Care Medicine Journal* states, "Mortality in sepsis is associated with the development of organ dysfunction. However, with the exception of corticosteroids for shock, specific therapies to reverse or prevent organ dysfunction remain unavailable."

Unfortunately, there is no more magic to do or to give today. No one knows what tomorrow holds, so we continue to work and HOPE!

Someone will come, and change will happen!

CHAPTER FIVE

Meet the Endothelial Glycocalyx and Sepsis, Who Live Together

Case Four: Heat stroke injury, presenting a sepsis-like course.

EMERGENCY! EMERGENCY! An Emergency transfer from the Boy Scout Camp was en route.

While they were transporting the patient, basic information was transmitted. He was a fifteen-year-old Boy Scout at a camp for the special needs scouts who were on a hike in the extremely hot sun. He was on the autism spectrum, and apparently, he did not like the water provided. He refused to drink and to follow the heat prevention measures that were provided.

Without warning, he collapsed. He was not sweating, had pale skin, and felt excessively hot. He remained unresponsive during the ambulance transport, but blood pressure and pulse remained satisfactory. His pulse was rapid with good perfusion.

His temperature initially was 108°F. Ice packs were applied to body and face, along with full exposure to air conditioning set at maximum to bring his temperature down during the transport.

On PICU arrival, he was comatose with rapid pupillary response to light but was otherwise unresponsive. The vital signs were blood pressure 128/75, pulse 160. He was cold in the areas covered by the ice bags, but otherwise warm. His general physical exam was quite unremarkable except for the deep comatose state.

The laboratory tests were only mildly abnormal, with an increased white blood cell count, hemoglobin at the upper normal limit, electrolytes were normal, the LDH was slightly increased. The urinalysis showed a specific gravity of 1.035, which is at the upper limit of normal.

Although he initially seemed stable, the ensuing hospital course was ALL DOWNHILL. He developed a disseminated intravascular coagulopathy with a very low platelet count, treated with platelet transfusions. He needed increased amounts of fluids to maintain urinary output, but even with large doses of diuretics, he retained large amounts of fluids.

He developed the MODS from the massive amounts of fluids required to maintain circulation and developed "third spacing" throughout his entire body. His respiratory status on full ventilator support steadily deteriorated following the ARDS disease progression.

Despite aggressive full supportive measures, his overall status continued to deteriorate. His abnormal neurological status (coma) remained unchanged but there were no neurologic signs to indicate brain death.

His downhill course continued with respiratory failure gradually becoming the most difficult aspect of his disease to manage. Ultimately, severe respiratory failure led to a cardiac arrest and death.

This was a case of heat stroke that presented a clinical disease pattern and course almost identical to sepsis and included the pattern of progressive organ failure. Heat stroke as the final diagnosis.

This case manifested clinical changes in a pattern similar to the changes seen in sepsis. Multi-organ failure, coagulopathy, inflammatory reactions, and third spacing; all developed in the absence of infection.

This unique case strongly suggests that many of the manifested problems seen in sepsis are a pattern of pathophysiologic dysfunction. This clinical problem was not compatible with the classic current definition of sepsis, as this patient did not have an infection-based insult but everything else was the same.

This is an important clinical observation of the pathophysiology of the human process of dying.

The Inflammatory cascade and the endothelial glycocalyx in the course of human disease, a discussion.

The **endothelial glycocalyx** (EGLX) is a major component of the inflammatory process. This chapter supplies an introduction and limited discussion of this extremely complex subject.

The EGLX was first recognized on the exterior surface of bacteria, and its role was explained as it was a means of "protection" for the bacteria from the external environment.

It took many years before glycocalyx was found within the human vascular system. The acceptance of the EGLX as an important constituent of the human vascular tree was recognized somewhat later.

The initial recognition of this glycocalyx physiologic benefit was the observation of the villi present on the luminal surface of the endothelial cells.

The first explanation given for the role of the glycocalyx was that the microvilli making up the brush border was for the protection of the body by a mechanism protecting from infection.

A further explanation was these microvilli that are electrically charged provided an electromagnetic force that prevented the circulating cells from making any contact with the vessel walls. These opposing electromagnetic forces cause the cells to essentially levitate, keeping the blood cells off the vessel walls. This mechanism creates an extremely low resistance within the circulatory system; the effect of electromagnetic forces. Therefore, there is extremely low resistance to the flow of the blood. The vascular system can function with low energy consumption to transport the blood components. This levitation effect keeps energy consumption to a very low portion of the cardiac workload. This allows plasma and the blood cells to be able to flow throughout the entire body while consuming very little energy.

That vascular resistance elimination feature alone justified the presence of the glycocalyx. This physiological role of the villi of the glycocalyx is accepted as an essential physiologic process.

For a while, the flow physiology was a very adequate explanation. This low resistance system is a remarkable physiologic biological engineering feat all by itself.

The continuing discoveries of additional physiologic effects contained within the EGLX presented an even more essential and much more complex role in human physiology.

The recent years of scientific basic research study have expanded the role of this "new organ." The glycocalyx has major additional roles in human physiology.

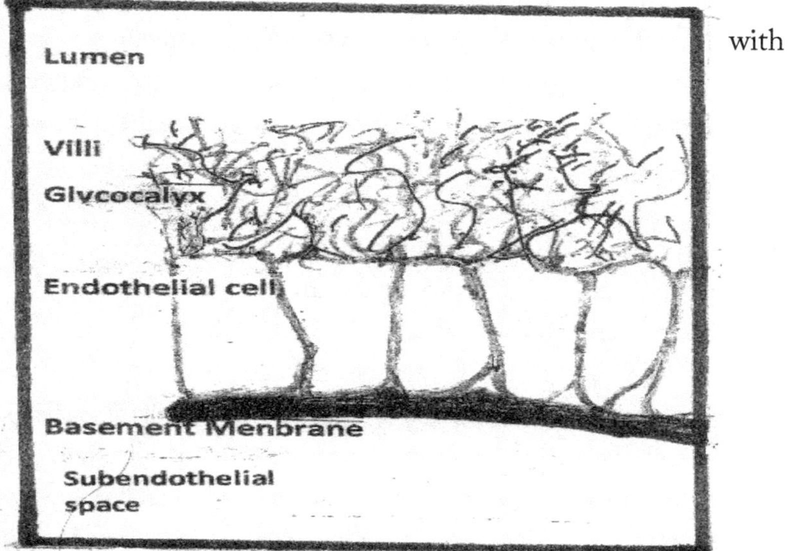

with

the vessel lumen at the top and the body tissue at the base.

The villi are clear on this drawing of a blood vessel. This is the vessel wall with the villi, the glycocalyx, endothelial cells, and the basement membrane clearly illustrated. The area where the endothelial cell base joins the basement membrane is shown. That basement membrane defines the margin of the subendothelial space. These areas play very important roles in this organ's function as clinically manifested.

The labelling of the structures clearly demonstrates the relationship of the key items: the villi, the glycocalyx, the endothelial cells, the basement membrane, and the subendothelial space. All have totally interdependent roles in the inflammatory response which is located within this structure.

The EGLX system is the largest organ system in the human body. This little known (and rarely discussed) organ system is an essential part of the human system. This human organ makes up the lining of the entire vascular system throughout the entire body.

Because the blood vessels have such an extensive network, especially when the capillary bed is included, the total area is huge, and the "organ" mass, although only single cell in depth, therefore is computed to be very large. The glycocalyx at this point is presumed to have the greatest mass of any organ in the human body. This means this EGLX is the largest organ of the human body. No quantitative mass calculation data for this newest organ has been included in the discussions.

The EGLX may not be uniformly distributed within the vascular system; some areas are thicker and others thinner. These inconsistencies make it impossible to precisely calculate the organ mass. The endothelial thickness varies by location within the vascular system and changes along the vessel's course to different values in different areas. Little precision accompanies this statement. The "measuring" process itself alters the thickness. These measurements are "old data" and should be qualitatively accepted.

This thickness variability creates problems for visualization and direct measurements using computerized visualization studies.

The age of the patient may also relate to thickness variability. As of today, the variance is not adequately explained, identified, or confirmed.

The work to define the glycocalyx structure has been extremely problematic. Any manipulation results in the destruction of the materials and loss of relationships. Furthermore, there is great difficulty in defining the structure. Then, even more problems are encountered when efforts are made to understand the specific physiologic functions present.

The glycocalyx is a very "hostile" region for scientific exploration.

More information is forthcoming as more sophisticated procedures are applied to the search. The thin, gel-like glycocalyx is exceedingly difficult to study; the glycocalyx just falls apart and all the structural relationships are lost. Studying the functions is even more problematic. This extreme difficulty is presented at every aspect of investigation. Progress is slow at best.

The metabolic and physiologic components all buried within the glycocalyx layer is the true picture of the glycocalyx organ, and those answers are slowly being worked out.

Deciphering this inflammatory process is much like solving a huge jigsaw puzzle. But this puzzle must be solved without the help of a picture, reference, operator's manual, or any other guidance. The final image or idea isn't even a concept yet. There is nothing to give any directions or help along to find an answer.

How many pieces will be needed to solve the puzzle?

No one has yet been able to describe this complicated system. Much of the basic data available is too limited and fragmented, and far too incomplete. Speculation upon the function always asks for more information. The data supplied makes the development of a more complete definition impossible now.

However, the beginning of the gross description and initial function is slowly starting to form. The greatest portion of the endothelial glycocalyx's role is still to be discovered and presented to the world.

Many chemical names and biological titles are presented in

unlinked investigative excerpts. This fragmented presentation makes the integration into a system still more problematic.

A source to begin a more in-depth review is a general literature review. This further research will provide more unrelated items at the forefront of medical discovery. You must match your personal needs and interests as the data are at best difficult.

Despite the newness of the research and the unequated complexity of the searches, a developing crude description of the inflammatory cascade can be crafted. These individual separate theories are, now, the best possible ideas. As new discoveries are made, certainly everything will be changed, updated, and hopefully clarified.

Many individual steps that are performed within glycocalyx are known, but the total pattern of the interdependence of these actions continues to confound everyone.

The many cytokines that are present are essential steps in the inflammatory cascade.

When a solution to a new single system of the cytokine system seems to be found, a clinical application is devised. A blocking agent or a facilitating agent is created. The novel application is applied. This cytokine and its function can now be confirmed. The techniques can facilitate or block the recently discovered function of the newly-recognized cytokine to define its function and clarify the role of this discovery. The use of a blocker and the facilitators should define the role and effect of that single system.

This is a time-tested and proven method to prove a system functions.

Too frequently these experiments, when applied to functions and cytokine systems within the glycocalyx, fail to achieve the full predicted effect. Some discoveries, while less than a total success, are still of value and some become a basis for new therapies. Many other trials show blind alleys that end and result in the elimination of exploration of that potential pathway.

The promising breakthrough benefit may be only partially realized.

The function is often best assessed through the use of antibodies or blocking chemicals. This frustrating difficult research must continue, and the development and implementation of theoretical potential solutions continue unabated.

When the EGLX "organ" is encountered in any way, the action of the observation alone often disrupts the structure, and that disorganization also compromises the glycocalyx function in addition to the visualization. Therefore, the creation of new and different techniques of study are needed to get any answers.

The researchers, if they are to move toward a new effective intervention in the treatment of inflammatory disease, must be able to access and analyze this unstable organ. The work to describe and understand EGLX functions will be difficult. Clarifying the EGLX characteristics is a large order, but it is getting done slowly now. It will become much more rapid as discoveries begin to happen. Almost miraculous technical breakthroughs are being presented and are to be applied to this problem.

Initially, all the attempts to define the human EGLX were failures. Even the measurements of glycocalyx thickness were different in different areas, and varying techniques added to the confusing picture. With more experience and better and different equipment, the scientific work of "knowing" the EGLX has slowly progressed. These studies supply information acquired through maximum difficulty over time from those researchers.

The function and physiologic dynamics of the EGLX are also being clarified in the same piecemeal manner as the structure. The progress is confusingly slow.

The description of the EGLX is both extremely complicated and essentially simple. The EGLX layer is composed of endothelial cells and their secreted products that make up the lining of the entire vascular system. The glycocalyx layer is a very thin layer covering all the interior luminal side of the vascular vessels including the arteries, veins, and capillaries. The analysis of structure and function is incredibly problematic.

The glycocalyx surface layer provides a low-resistance interface between the endothelial cells and the blood cells within the circulation based on the functions of the microvilli.

The surface below the villi initially seemed to be a gel, but the real surface is actually made up of all intertwined filaments originating from the endothelial cells.

The glycocalyx layer maintains an electromagnetic charge, and the circulating cells maintain an opposing electromagnetic charge. This situation therefore creates a levitation-like separation between the endothelial cells and the plasma proteins and circulating blood cells.

Does the elimination of this levitation effect allowing the blood cells to contact the deeper structures of the glycocalyx actually start the cytokine cascade? This loss of levitation as an inciting factor seems to be a likely mechanism that starts the cascade.

The importance of this very low-resistance border cannot be underappreciated as the physiologic impact is considered. Where, if anywhere, does this electromagnetic originate, and does this relate to the cytokine activation portion of the glycocalyx system? Is this the mechanical dysfunction that incites the cytokine activities? Is the disease onset related to loss of the levitation factor?

This small physical separation eliminates the resistance to flow and allows unimpeded blood flow even through the tiniest capillaries. The cells in a healthy blood vessel do not have contact with the vessel wall at any point in the passage. The presence of this low resistance is needed to allow the circulatory system to work effectively.

This electromechanical force is strong enough to distort the RBC's configuration during their capillary passage. This nearly complete elimination of vessel wall flow resistance is an extremely important issue and initially seemed to be the entire role for the presence of the endothelial glycocalyx.

But there is so much more! The EGLX is an extremely dynamic structure that provides far more essential functions than the hydraulic viscosity support. While the viscosity miracle is so important, the lower layer of metabolic cytokines and their endothelial cells have a functional complexity even more essential in the pathophysiologic function of the inflammatory response.

The endothelial cells and their secretions make up the "gel-like" layer on the intravascular side of the vessels. In reality, this "gel" is the surface of the glycoprotein interface of the many different individual strands. This glycocalyx "gel" includes many important and widely different physiologic functions. Certainly, at this time, all this endothelial glycocalyx's functions are not known or listed and are definitely not understood.

Known physiologic functions are:

1. Controlling the third spacing of fluids into the extracellular space.
2. Supporting the cardiac function with vasoactive support and fluid volume control
3. Activation of the platelet response to injury with agglutination and coagulation system activation
4. Stimulation of the macrocytes and activation of immune cellular response
5. Coagulation control of blood clotting and blood clot lysis regulation both in normal and disease conditions
6. Blood-brain barrier permeability regulation to control fluids and metabolic products separate from vascular control
7. Vascular dilation and participation in blood pressure control
8. Many more physiologic modulating activities yet to be defined

These listed actions are all very gross actions and easily observed, but certainly additional countless small important actions will be discovered within this defensive organ or homeostatic organ system. How should the EGLX be described?

The control of the microcirculation is one highly active essential function of the EGLX. The endothelial cells and the accompanying glycocalyx control the mechanical transduction needed to adjust the blood pressure. Control of the vascular permeability seems to be located at the same site. This mechanical transduction action is related to intrinsic nitrous oxide metabolic interactions. This means vascular vasodilation control is partially within the endothelial glycocalyx. The nitrous oxide system is the chemical mediator of blood pressure.

How does the nitrous oxide system relate to the sympathetic nervous system? Where do the adrenergic stimulant drugs act? Even with some some knowledge of blood pressure control and fluid, all known data presents a confusing relationship that eventually controls vasoconstriction and vasodilation function.

There is so much more to be learned about the mechanisms of circulatory control. Both locally controlled vessels and the sympathetic nervous system blood pressure control input are actively involved in blood pressure control. How does each component get its input into the control of the vascular system? Where do the catecholamines fit into this game? Where do vasoconstrictors fit and how do they act?

How and why do the vasodilators actually work? They do work and do play a vital role in the treatment of hypotension in septic shock.

Injury to the glycocalyx leads to vascular permeability with loss of control of extravasation of fluid into the extracellular space. The fluid control mechanism is yet unclear but is far more complex than the Starling Law of the Capillary[1] originally proposed, which states: fluid movement between blood and tissues is determined by differences in hydrostatic and colloid osmotic (oncotic) pressures between plasma inside the microvessels and fluid outside in the extracellular space.

Severe injury to the endothelial cells allows the intracellular space

---

1   CC Michel, TE Woodcock, FE Curry, "Understanding and Extending the Starling Principle." *Acta Anaesthesiologica Scandinavica.* U.S. National Library of Medicine. Accessed March 9, 2023. https://pubmed.ncbi.nlm.nih.gov/32270491/#:~:text=The%20Starling%20Principle%20states%20that,microvessels%20and%20fluid%20outside%20them.

to enlarge by accepting the albumin and fluids that leave the systemic circulation and compound the vasodilatory shock component of septic shock syndrome.

Fluid loss seems to correlate with a very severe injury. The endothelial intracellular pore transduction of fluids is probably related to endothelial cellular injury that results in cell function paralyses, or cell death. The intracellular spaces between the cells are open and the basement membrane "pores" do not stop the rapid fluid equilibration between the vascular space and the subendothelial space. This fluid flux causes a secondary hypovolemic state.

Knowledge of the relationships of the endothelial cells with the production and control of the proteoglycans has been described. The proteoglycan production and maintenance in response to injury to the endothelial cells have barely been described.

Even the time for recovery of endothelial cell repairs is largely an estimate and currently is measured in days. Too little information is known about the glycocalyx regeneration process.

The extensive fluid shift along with active vasodilation causes the recognized clinical problem of hypovolemia and vasodilation related shock. These physical measurements of patient physiology are the hallmark of septic shock in its clinical presentation.

So many more essential functions still need clarification and expansion.

The vessel lining is again illustrated here. A villous border is shown and the distance between the cells and the vessel wall is related to the electric charge creating a force keeping the cells away from the villi of the endothelial cells. The deeper structures are poorly defined and are the site of the metabolically active systems leading to the development of the cytokine storm.

The structure of the glycocalyx is poorly defined and seems for now a result of random construction. Currently, there is no known formatted defined structural skeleton. No standardized proteoglycan has been found to have a consistent interactive controlling relationship with any other proteoglycans to form a structure.

While this undefined gel-like structure is the current descriptive experience for endothelial glycocalyx, other physiologic experiences show that most structures do have relatively set relationships to their surrounding structures. Establishing this relationship clarification is a goal for the future.

The impression that the glycocalyx is a complex interwoven layer may not be correct. The glycocalyx layers seem to be more like spaghetti than feathers, but who really knows. The glycocalyx is such a vital area of semi-known products, and all these products seem very metabolically active.

This drawing is being shown again to demonstrate the relationships of the EGLX components.

The initial proteoglycan layer is secreted by the endothelial cells and seems to keep its continuity with the originating mother cell. These proteoglycans are secreted by and remain anchored to the endothelial cell. Each proteoglycan passes through the transmembrane dome of the protein core and spreads out into the matrix. These varied proteoglycans are presumed to supply a soft supportive skeleton in which the glycosaminoglycan chains are supported and intermingled in a presumed random manner.

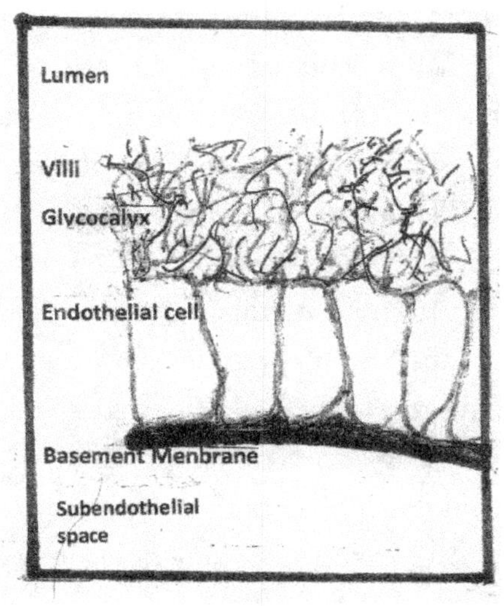

Albumin included within the EGLX is measured and is a significant part of this glycocalyx layer. The role and origin of the albumin and its position and functional role in this matrix are yet to be elucidated. As of now, it is just considered to be present. Albumin is a chemically and enzymatically inactive product so the role it plays is not clear. The role of the albumin may be that of a buffer separating active functions or keeping the reactions from activating. The quantity of albumin may vary for an unknown number of reasons. None of these concepts attribute an active role to albumin.

This product list of the glycocalyx consists of many varied entities, including the heparin sulfate proteoglycans (e.g., glypicans, perlecans, and syndecans). The glycosaminoglycan compounds are heparan sulfate and chondroitin sulfate, dermatan sulfate, keratin sulfate, and others. Hyaluronan (hyaluronic acid) is a neutral compound and inter-reacts with other glycosaminoglycans to form the gel-like material that "stabilizes" the structure, and the gel layer retains water.

Many isolated reports of new and different compounds and the possible actions are presented but this new data initially is difficult to integrate into the "scheme of things" within the glycocalyx.

Hyaluronan is synthesized and degraded at the rate of five grams per day. So many products are acting and reacting constantly in this surprisingly metabolic region. Defining the responsibility of each component involved and in what manner that activity takes place will have to eventually be defined. These discoveries will be a part of under-standing and clarifying the cure. More details of other components could also be listed but, at least now, would only add to the puzzle.

But that is not the whole story of the glycocalyx. The content and structure of this layer is extraordinarily complex and, worse yet, very dynamic. Even more miracles hide in this "organ." Persistence and time will bring the answers to us.

You will see it when you believe it! Or maybe believe it to see it! It is discovery in action.

CHAPTER SIX

The Endothelial Glycocalyx (EGLX)

Case Five: Inflammation and sepsis from burns

The day started as a lovely July summer day. The loveliness ended when a twelve-year-old boy came into the PICU.

He had brought lunch out to his father working in the field. They were baling hay for their cattle. After their lunch was finished, the tractor was restarted, igniting a gasoline fume explosion. Gasoline had leaked out of the carburetor system and evaporated. This highly explosive gas just pooled in the small depression at the edge of the open field. The adults were taller and sustained only minor injuries. The boy was much shorter and was totally encompassed in the blast site.

He sustained 42 percent burns over his exposed body and also had a serious respiratory tree burn injury.

Management followed the established burn treatment protocols. Sedation and analgesia were immediately provided for his pain management; the initial burn management. He was immediately intubated to protect his upper and lower airway from presumed airway burn. He was placed on controlled ventilation using analgesics and sedation. He tolerated all the sedations and the burn cares well.

He was stable on the PICU care routines and was kept comfortable on the sedation analgesic medications. The burn fluid volumes were standard, and these intravenous fluids maintained the urinary output.

His mother (an RN) stayed at his bedside, continuously providing loving support. The plan was to continue the sedation for the first seventy-two hours (about three days) and then reassess his airway and pulmonary status. It was expected he would be a candidate for extubation.

His course could not have been simpler or more straightforward since all parameters were physiologic.

But on the fourth morning, when his sedation routine was weaned as per protocol, he had absolutely no response!

Nothing had happened, nothing at all, but the neurologic exam showed brain death.

The monitor recordings were reviewed, and the mother had stayed at the bedside all night. The nurses and staff noted no changes during the care throughout the night, nothing unusual had happened, but he was certainly dead anyhow. This was a silent brain death (totally unexplained).

Actress Ann Hecht seems to have had the same process happen to her, dead after an apparently moderate burn injury. She had been responding well to the burn treatment but developed unexplained brain death. (Information from the 2022 media reports only).

Sometimes the answers cannot be found. There was nothing to be done differently. No changes to make things better.

Worst of all, no answers for anyone, especially the family and the doctor.

Burns cause inflammation and the inflammatory cascade occurs; was that the answer? Perhaps someday an explanation will be found.

It is so hard to try to save a life, and then fail, and then not to get any answers That is the worst!

More on the endothelial glycocalyx functions

No attempt is made or even will be made to clarify or to integrate the functions of the glycocalyx here. The subject will basically be listed and briefly discussed, but no integrated function can be projected to explain anything about this case here.

In an abstract concept, the glycocalyx seems like a huge jigsaw puzzle with an unknown number of pieces and many pieces not yet found. What will the answer be like? Incidentally, no "picture" of the end result can even be suggested by even the most knowledgeable.

Sepsis is the result of an inflammatory response to injury to the endothelial glycocalyx. The accepted definition of sepsis still varies a little and is an enduring source of discussion. The conclusion generally is the same, but the vocabulary often varies.

In the June 2022 issue of *Critical Care Medicine,* two unrelated articles provided slightly different sepsis definitions. These are physiologically equivalent in the final conclusion, but the different wording shows the persisting dynamic changes are still at work.

The pathophysiologic problems active in sepsis originate largely in the EGLX site. Endothelial dysfunction and glycocalyx damage are active responses to problems created by any form of injury.

These complicated physiologic responses vary and even change during the course of "sepsis illness." The poorly defined "injury" occurs and persists and changes the physiologic responses over time, and the "illness" progresses to manifest the problems of sepsis. This creates definition and recognition issues.

This observation that new components of the "illness" manifest after the initial presentation is a common course during sepsis. This variation in disease course was initially noted by Semmelweis. At times, this variation is so marked that a different medical condition is believed to be the cause of the illness.

The EGLX layer is clearly damaged, and this "damage" contributes to some aspect or aspects of the inflammatory cascade that clinically presents as sepsis.

Chemical components of the EGLX layer are found circulating within the blood when sepsis occurs. However, these breakdown products that are released from the EGLX do not define a chemical diagnosis of sepsis. The concentrations and patterns of different chemicals and timing of the release from the glycocalyx do not allow a laboratory diagnosis of sepsis. Although it seems intuitive, the prediction of the severity of the sepsis does not correlate in any manner either.

Very active research efforts are currently underway and hopefully will soon provide a definitive answer to whether this is sepsis. Clinically this will be so helpful.

Chemical components derived from the basic glycocalyx components are released during sepsis, showing that glycocalyx damage is a generic response. The pattern and volume of the individual specific products released from the glycocalyx currently do not define the physiologic dysfunction, nor do they define the type of disease manifestation, nor do they clarify the diagnosis of the sepsis disease state present. They only show EGLX injury.

Genetic components seemed to be predictive of sepsis, but in the end, there is still no answer.

Multiple clinically recognizable manifestations of sepsis are directly attributed to the complex systems that make up this dynamic body organ. Clinical problems can be correlated with activation of some components of the glycocalyx but are not specific enough. Location or type of injury may be similar, but each disease presentation is unique in its manifestation or may be the same.

Dynamic changes in the EGLX system are generally a part of the sepsis syndrome. An ever-changing clinical disease presentation is a hallmark of sepsis pathology.

The protective glycocalyx villus layer becomes damaged, and due to its very fragile and unstable characteristics, is essentially removed and the vessels are left with a bare surface to make direct contact with the cell walls of the component cells of the blood. This is most likely the mechanism of injury.

Platelet and leukocyte seem to have direct contact with the glycocalyx and the endothelial cells after the villi are gone. These altered vessel components allow direct platelet and cell contact with the deeper glycocalyx or endothelial cell layers. This contact causes platelets and white cells to start rolling, which brings into activation the ICAM-1 and VCAM-1 systems. This modification of white blood cells leads to neutrophil adherence and clustering. Platelet adherence results in increased platelet adhesiveness, leading to platelet masses. The white cells activate and migrate from within the intravascular space into the surrounding tissues. This is the start of the continuing cellular inflammatory response in the tissues. This is a response that may extinct rapidly to nothing, or it may progress to become severe sepsis syndrome.

Clinically petechiae are the earliest presentation of platelet activation. The laboratory correlation is a drop in the platelet count to abnormally low levels. Bleeding from thrombocytopenic (low platelet count) is quite variable from patient to patient. These aggregated platelets may be causing thrombosis and preventing blood flow to the damaged area, ending the risk to the host. Alternatively, this activated platelet may continue the cellular inflammatory response.

An undefined glycocalyces injury creates a coagulation pathology. Glycocalyx activation leads to intravascular thrombosis and thrombin system (the secondary clot lysis system) is activated creating very dynamic interactions (clotting and lysis occurring almost simultaneously), clinically manifesting as Disseminated Intravascular Coagulopathy (DIC). Acute arterial thrombosis leads to limb loss. Inability to clot leads to massive hemorrhage and skin manifestations of purpura (purple color of the skin). These are disastrous complications of the "sepsis syndrome." This is only one of many dysfunctional problems.

Each factor definitely has a role which still needs clarification. Thrombosis and clot lysis is the pattern of disseminated intravascular coagulopathy. Both the thrombotic and the coagulopathy activities originate within the glycocalyx. The clotting cascade and its multiple factors are well defined, but the relationship within the glycocalyx during activation has yet to be clarified.

Von Willebrand factor is also a component within the glycocalyx and plays a unique and different role in coagulopathy of sepsis. This activity is somehow different than DIC. The where and how this interaction occurs will need to be explained. Will some related aspect of the Von Willebrand system become a bleeding treatment factor?

To anti-coagulate or not to anti-coagulate; that is the clinical problem! Coagulation and bleeding are big-time clinical problems and will not to be addressed here. Clinically, there are multiple approaches to be used as the problems manifest differently. Supportive measures are generally used, blood transfusion being the most frequent, but fresh never frozen plasma less than five days old adds something more to the system that is not present in older or previously frozen plasma. But in less than fresh never frozen plasma, clotting factors can be measured and directly replaced to control bleeding.

Sometimes just watching seems to be the best course.

The platelet activation also contributes to coagulation problems. This coagulation cascade is well documented in clinical situations. The activation begins at the I-CAM-1 and the V CAM-1 published scientific descriptions. This physiologic process discussion will not be repeated here.

The lymphocytes join into the cell activation pattern and provide anti-infective forces for host protection in coordination with the immune system activation. Antigen recognition and template manufacture and retention of recognition is another complex macrocyte response that happens here in this interrelated process. Macrocyte response and antibody production does not happen within the glycocalyx organ but is a part of the lymphatic system. There are more complete discussions of this physiologic process in the bibliography.

The lymphocytes and the histiocyte cells have been associated with the hemophagocytic lymphohistiocytosis syndrome (HLH) and are the mechanism involved in the cytokine storm response. Interleukin-2 receptors are markedly elevated. A specific antibody product was designed and produced with properties that blocked the specific interleukin response need name of the cytokine and the antigen used. But the disease (HLH) persisted despite the documentation of highly effective binding of this specific interleukin. The diagnosis is supported by elevated ferritin levels (a product related to hemoglobin production). Where ferritin fits into this process has yet to be clarified.

TNF alpha clearly has roles in autoimmune diseases and the products are seen in multiple television advertisements in the USA. Interleukin 3 (IL-3) is linked to a disease condition of polymyalgia rheumatica, an autoimmune disease-causing pain and joint restriction. This condition responds to corticosteroids. Many new effective products are now available for specific autoimmune related diseases because of these extremely complex difficult research work.

Interleuken-6 is the cause of fever with infection and happens very early in the disease process.

The answer to this problem of interleukin- and cytokine-created problems is predicted by specific treatment with antibodies specific to that cytokine, which supplies only partial control and blockage. Some portions of the basic problem persist. The failure of a specifically designed agent is confounding and confusing.

Why does it not work like it should? What more is here that we don't know?

Cytokine adsorption technique has been used for removal of the toxic components found in the blood. The cytokine absorption columns have repeatedly failed to control the problems of the sepsis disease state. Absorbing the toxins (poisons) and removing them all from the bloodstream is a great theory. These complicated clinical procedures were performed with exceptional execution, but this technique did not result in a disease or sepsis cure. Something more seems to be happening, but what?

Far better explanations of individual actions and drug trials are available for review in the general literature than are presented here.

Shock is a major manifestation and is difficult to manage and correlates with mortality. This too is a complex interaction of so many components.

Capillary leakage and endothelial cell damage play a major undefined role.

Vascular relaxation was discovered to be regulated by nitrous oxide metabolism, and this discovery was rewarded with a Nobel Prize for Medicine.

The activation of nitric oxide synthase allows the release of nitric oxide (which causes vasodilation) within the glycocalyx. Nitrous oxide release relaxes the vascular tone and increases the size of the vascular space, which decreases blood pressure. These vascular tone changes cause a clinically measurable decrease in systemic blood pressure. These measured changes are due to vessel dilation, and in the active disease state, the hypovolemia is worsened by extracellular fluid loss.

The intravascular fluids leave the severely damaged EGLX and move to the extra cellular space. Once the endothelial cells are damaged, the spaces between the endothelial cells (formerly called pores) are now wide open and allow free fluid movement out of the circulation leading to hypotension and shock. The endothelial cells are either "paralyzed" or dead. Vasoactive medications can increase blood pressure and improve circulation but have no effect on the "third spacing syndrome" fluid shifts.

The effects of various unspecified metabolites are implicated in the process of healing and support neovascularization and many other inflammation healing responses. Who? What? And when? More to come!

Many of the metabolized products are involved in the directed cellular migration process of the macrophages and the lymphocytes and manifest the immune system's cellular response. These are the same cells that are also included in the creation of autoimmune related diseases and hemophagocytic lymphohistiocytosis. Interferon and Interleukin 18, interferon-3, and TNF alpha are also part of this cytokine release pathology. These interactions are difficult to describe. Descriptions of these interactions are alluded to in the studies, but further clarification will be coming soon.

Proinflammatory cytokines are released, and these unusual compounds may activate heparinase 1 and other cytokines that are usually inactive enzymes. Heparinase 1 is broken down into subunits resulting in a 65 k Dalton to 8 k Dalton and 50 k Dalton subunits that form the physiologically active enzyme heparinase.

This metabolic modification of heparinase-1 into various products is associated with Damage Associated Molecular Activity (DAMPS). This inflammatory response is also produced by live cells that are injured. DAMPS is also released from dead and dying cells particularly as a pattern of cellular necrosis. Cellular death with necrosis causes an intense activation of the inflammatory process. TNF alpha is only one of many chemical products released from dead and dying cells.

What the role of other newly discovered processes of cell death is only speculation.

Many less well described functions occur when this action-packed layer is activated. More things are happening here than have been detailed in the general reports.

These initial actions are only the tip of the iceberg in this unbelievably complex system involved in the act of dying at the cellular level. It seems only to get more complicated as more becomes known. Where do these individual puzzle pieces begin to fit?

The standardized animal models of sepsis used generally start with induction by lipopolysaccharide infusion; these models demonstrate glycocalyx damage and vascular permeability. The release of biomarkers such as syndecan-1 release confirms the scientific premise that EGLX destruction occurs during the sepsis syndrome.

A great deal of the research on sepsis uses the established experimental model for the studies. The liposaccharide experimental induction of the sepsis syndrome is very intense stimulus. This particular means of inducing the signs and pathology of sepsis may cause a response that is so intensely destructive that individual patterns of disease and disease progression cannot be defined. This excessive damage response by the test model may invalidate many of the studies of sepsis. Even this consideration causes a reconsideration of the data already presented.

Cell death causes TNF alpha release and is a very potent pathological process that causes other cell death and accelerates an unlimited inflammatory cascade. These GCLX breakdown products are some of the agents used in the research of sepsis in animals.

The research with varying products to induce and recreate disease patterns provides a confusing pattern of illness and patterns with significant variability. All these variable responses make conclusions from induced models of sepsis quite difficult.

Shock is a major part of sepsis. Fluid therapy is the primary treatment of sepsis. Septic shock and circulatory failure occur currently and are attributed to the third spacing syndrome. The shock state is due to the combination of capillary leakage and vascular space dilatation. The shock has elements of both vascular space enlargement and fluid extravasation into the extracellular tissues.

Edema (leading to anasarca) and massive fluid overload are common late phase manifestations of the sepsis syndrome and easily recognized but are present only after the shock is aggressively treated. Volume replacement with albumin seems to be only slightly more beneficial than replacement with crystalloids (saline solutions) or other volume replacement products, but the same complications third spacing of fluids into the extracellular space happen with all.

Starling's Law of the Capillary has for more than a century supplied guidance during the consideration of fluid dynamics. This physiologic principle expressed has been generally accepted, but when reviewed in 2012, the Starling Principle rules did not explain the observed dynamics. When the glycocalyx as factor is considered, a vastly different dynamic is present. Starling's law no longer provides any explanation for fluid flux and physiologic changes. This review of Starling's law can be as simple or complex as the observer desires, but at this point Starling's principle is only an interesting historical model.

A huge amount of early sepsis research largely focused on the problem of circulatory failure and fluid dynamics. Severe capillary dilation requires increased circulating volumes to support a full vascular system. Extracellular fluid loss into the extracellular space compounds the problem.

Sepsis management protocols for fluid replacement have been developed to minimize the problems of third spacing. These recommendations are revised frequently.

The action of catecholamines on this dilated vascularity are mediated via the sympathetic nervous system, but the interaction of the cellular nitrous oxide and the sympathetic nervous system have yet to be described. Despite the lack of explanation, the clinical application of catecholamines supplies an effective pharmacologic means of circulatory support during the clinical approach to sepsis management.

Fluid replacement programming has a major beneficial contribution to sepsis treatment. These resuscitation protocols often rapidly infuse massive amounts of crystalloid, but this aggressive fluid treatment has led to the development MODS, which is a new diagnosis developed in concordance with Critical Care Medical Specialty development. The most recent fluid revamping was published in the *New England Journal of Medicine* in June 2022. Changes recommended were relatively small and primarily addressed the chemistry of the fluid.

This massive fluid shift causes organ dysfunction and failure, and when unchecked leads to death, as the sepsis syndrome does not stop. Survival statistics clearly show better survival with the early aggressive fluid regimens when compared to the period prior to using effective fluid resuscitation.

But these interventions do not end the fluid management problems. The large amounts of fluids seem to compromise organ function and can lead to organ failure. Autopsy studies show severe edema and increase spacing of the cells of the organs.

But there is much more to sepsis syndrome than circulatory failure. Coagulopathy is an important aspect. This is most commonly seen as disseminated intravascular coagulopathy (DIC). Clotting and clot lysis follows. The products of fibrinolysis are present and interfere with clotting. Low fibrinogen levels result and further interfere with coagulation. During the Covid-19 pandemic thrombosis was a problem and anticoagulation protocols were developed and used. The coagulopathy and the low platelet count levels contribute to the bleeding problems.

The inflammatory and cellular responses cause fever and perpetuate the cellular reaction.

A large number of metabolically active compounds are included in the glycocalyx complex. Each individual component has a different role and its own pattern of action.

These chemical products that are known today can be listed, but certainly this is not a complete inventory. The apparent functions of these components are listed reflecting what is assumed today, and the patterns of interaction are yet to be determined. The list is quite incomplete, and new discoveries, modifications, and expansions certainly will be found.

Even the interactions and actions, even though more than speculation, are far from clearly defined metabolic patterns with specific actions. To even suggest how these products interact to provide support for the purpose of repairing glycocalyx cannot be entertained today with the information available.

How important is the process of separation of the blood components from interacting with the glycocalyx? What causes damage to the vascular wall? This type of injury apparently allows the whole cytokine activation process to start and to continue. This explanation is only speculation now.

How and what is the role of the glycocalyx barrier in keeping pathogens out of the system, and if so, how does that protective action happen? The barrier function of the glycocalyx is presumed to be present and supply a beneficial function, similar to the way that the glycocalyx layer on the bacterial cell wall protects the bacteria from attack.

So much is still unknown about the various functions and roles of this critical body organ, the glycocalyx.

Each review results in even more questions. So many important questions are without answers today, but these answers will be forthcoming as a new increased research focus on the glycocalyx is developing.

More data and incomplete conclusions about the EGLX are presented in the next several paragraphs.

This presentation provides poorly organized, confusing lists of materials. This list may be just an inventory listing of some but not all components of the glycocalyx.

Here are the semi-detailed descriptions of some of the known components of the glycocalyx:

The EGLX is a villous layer consisting of a polysaccharide protein composite structure found on the apical membrane of the endothelial cells of the vascular system. The location places it between the blood vessel wall and the circulating plasma, decreasing the "vascular work" of circulating cells through such small vessels. The red blood cells must deform to pass through the capillary bed. This further shows the effect of the negative charges in the separation mechanically to avoid contact and stress. What is the role of the endothelial cells in creating or supporting this electromagnetic force? Does the loss of this force allow the collapse of the glycocalyx and the unleashing of the cytokine storm? Little to no data about this portion of this functioning system is available.

The glycocalyx layer contains glycoproteins, proteoglycans, and glycosaminoglycans directly originating from the surface of the endothelial cells. This glycocalyx completely covers the entire luminal surface of the vascular endothelium. Many other chemical compounds are also present within the glycocalyx and are yet to be defined as dynamic actors in the function and also dysfunction of this organ.

The glycocalyx component list includes glycoproteins, proteoglycans, glycosaminoglycans (GAGs), cell surface receptors (selectins and integrins), hyaluronic acids, albumin, and other metabolic components of these basic products and others not yet discovered. The supra-endothelial region of the glycocalyx is a much denser region and therefore studies become more problematic. To be able to define compounds and also assess function is a heroic task.

Members of the immunoglobulin superfamily with sialic acid residuals and oligosaccharide chains attached are present within the glycocalyx.

Versican and perlecan, with their adsorbed plasma proteins, e.g., albumin and orosomucoid, add to the density of supra-endothelial region. At the apical surface of the endothelial cell membranes are the GAG families; heparan sulfate (HS), hyaluronic acid (HA), and chondroitin dermatan sulfate (CS) are in this mix.

The core proteoglycans are transmembrane syndecans that seem to maintain the endothelial cell membrane connection. The endothelial cell is anchored by glypicans and associated perlecan to provide extensions into the glycocalyx. The inferior wall of the cell membrane is attached to the basement membrane. Hyaluronic acid binds to the transmembrane CD44 proteins. The syndecans and the CD4 are part of the cytoskeleton's organization which are attached to the cortical actin framework of the reticuloendothelial system within the cell. The glypicans bind to the cell membrane.

This pattern of molecular structure seems to be consistent in the healthy glycocalyx structure at the capillary level. Different glycocalyx composition patterns seem to exist in different organs. The glycocalyx pattern is different during pathological conditions.

The thickness of the glycocalyx could be related to its protective role. Low serum albumin levels and thinner glycocalyx layers seem to relate to worse inflammatory responses to infection. Could this be a predictor of severe disease? Time will tell!

The foregoing listing was included to show the complexity and exemplify our incomplete definition and understanding of this complex medical organ.

No attempt is made or even will be made to clarify or to integrate the functions of the glycocalyx subject in this presentation. So many linkages and bridges do not seem to be in place, so relationships seem to be mere speculation.

In concept, the glycocalyx seems like a huge jigsaw puzzle with an unknown number of pieces, and with so many pieces not yet found. What will the answer be like? Incidentally, no "picture" of the end result can even be suggested. Create the pattern within your mind.

Please refer to the review article that begins a presentation of the Glycocalyx.

Some very complex functions are found within the glycocalyx, and some will be presented as these functions are presumed to be somewhat understood based upon published papers.

Vascular Integrity Control: The EGLX is an endothelial barrier. The EGLX regulates vascular permeability, renal proteinuria, vasodilatation, and leukocyte and platelet adhesion. The heparan sulfate S proteoglycans regulate many of these functions. All the components synergize actions to maintain the vascular integrity and provide organ protection health. The glycocalyx and the endothelial cells both contribute actively to the maintenance of an intact vascular barrier.

Shear Stress Transmission (e.g., blood pressure control): Evidence is accumulating that the EGLX is involved in the wall mediated by shear stress responses. The exact mechanism remains unclear. The specific connections of the core proteins to the actin cytoskeleton (the syndecans) and the plasma membrane (the glypicans) seem to mediate intracellular signaling for nitrous oxide production. But there is so much more complex physiology to be discovered and to be clarified for us all.

Vascular Homeostasis Modulation: Vascular homeostasis is modulated through the physical barrier properties of the glycocalyx and the endothelial cells. A thinner glycocalyx is associated with increased leukocyte endothelial interaction. Metalloproteases (MMP7) is a proteinase that specifically cleaves syndecan-1 (SDC-1) and in the studies of platelet adhesion SDC-1 was increased. Glycocalyx degradation correlates with monocyte-endothelial adhesion, plasminogen activator inhibitor-1 and intercellularmolecule-1 ICAM-1) release. The EGLX certainly plays a key role in the regulation of vascular inflammatory response and blood clotting functions.

Conditions for EGLX dysfunction are not known:

When the balance of EGLX degradation (thinning) occurs and the restitution is disturbed, a disease state is present. Resolution of the glycocalyx to normal presumes the end of the disease state.

This list of pathological conditions is not complete, but the similarity of their disease presentation strongly suggests a basic functional disturbance is common to all physiologic dysfunctions.

Medical conditions that result in EGLX changes include infection, sepsis, trauma, inflammation, ischemia-reperfusion injury, shock hyperthermia, hypervolemia, hypertension, hypoxia, hypernatremia, hyperglycemia, and diabetes and atherosclerosis, and certainly other diseases and more conditions not yet identified.

Sepsis and trauma are allies in triggering the Inflammatory process: Degradation of the EGLX occurs also in non-infective inflammation responses that includes trauma.

Tumor necrosis factor (TNF-alpha) that results after heparinase cleaves TNF alpha is a major proinflammatory cytokine early in the inflammatory cascade.

Circulating SDC-1 in high concentrations serves as a marker of EGLX shedding and is seen in trauma. SDC-1 is associated with sympathomimetic activation, inflammation, tissue injury, and mortality in initial reports. This product is not a diagnostic or predictor of sepsis. Developmental work on a diagnostic product is underway.

Preservation of the EGLX effectively suppresses ICAM-1 and VCAM-1- E-selectin is found in response to TNF alpha. This response pattern dampens the proinflammatory cytokines release and slows the progress of the inflammation.

Blockage of TNF alpha in theory should stop or slow sepsis. But when the antigen was clinically applied, very little clinical improvement was noted. Other antibodies to Il-6 and other products promoting inflammatory diseases have been disappointing. Repeated attempts to create and apply antibody blockage of Il-6 and other specific proinflammatory compounds have been failures, but this area still seems promising and related products are being manufactured and tested.

Fibroblast growth factor receptor-1(FGFR-1) and HS biosynthetic enzyme Exostatin 1 (EXT1) both support the repair or regeneration of the glycocalyx. However, the FGFR/EXT 1 (fibroblast growth factor pathway and the exostatin pathway) are inhibited in sepsis. This observation supports the idea that this pathway contributes to the preservation or recovery of the glycocalyx. However, as is so common in these glycocalyx studies, the complete blockage of FGFR/EXT 1 pathway does not suppress recovery. This shows that some other pathways also support restoration of the glycocalyx.

The pattern and factors influencing the restoration of the glycocalyx are also very unclear. There is only a limited amount of data available for consideration. The understanding of the restoration process of the glycocalyx will be an important step in the development of products to support this metabolic process.

The recovery or repair of the EGLX in-vivo is estimated to take five to seven days. Even this seemingly simple observation has provided only estimates in days.

The data about the EGLX is presented in these confusing piecemeal patterns. The mixed facts and very incomplete presentations make the basis for large presumptions that must fill the gaps in knowledge.

This is "the current state of the art." Even some of the data may not be complete or even accurate, as that is the state of a constant investigation into this very complicated system.

The problems associated with the highly unstable fragile nature of the EGLX structure results in uncertainty. When even the determination of separating the normal from the damaged EGLX is unclear, so many items must be defined, which makes this analytic work extremely challenging. The fragility of the EGLX severely compromises every attempt to analyze the compounds and is especially more difficult when trying to determine the function of the subunits studied.

Each analysis becomes so complex that only the most dedicated, experienced researchers with extensive resources can even consider the study of intensely complex products. This EGLX research seems to be a case of low immediate return on investment of scarce resources.

Finding a product that provides an active role in stopping sepsis, or even modifying the glycocalyx dysfunction of the inflammatory process, shall eventually point to a solution. This will increase the numbers of researchers and the number of scientific studies will accelerate.

This brief discussion of the glycocalyx should not be considered a primer or roadmap through this amazing subject, only a very incomplete introduction.

So very much is left to know about the role of the glycocalyx in health and disease.

Even the factors facilitating recovery from a disease process (sepsis) that must occur to have sepsis survivors, also remains a near total mystery.

However, this compromised limited knowledge base is what we have today, and this points toward where the answer lies!

This indeed is the great SEPSIS GOLD MINE of the future scientific research.

CHAPTER SEVEN

What is Sepsis, Really?

Case Six: Ready to die

A man presented himself to the emergency department in a strange and unusual manner. When asked why he came, he said, "I came at the request of my family. I told them to come home as I was dying and wanted to see them all. The whole family reacted and demanded that I come in and get treated, and here am. I am sorry to put you through it."

He was a well-dressed courteous gentleman in his late seventies. His initial vital signs were normal. The general physical exam was quite unremarkable.

When he was informed that no disease state was found, He re-emphasized that he was just beginning to die, and the process would become clearer soon. Because he was so adamant and the family was equally firm, he was admitted for observation.

The whole battery of admission tests were all within the normal range. The chest X-ray did not show a tumor in his chest. The EKG showed only non-specific ST-T changes.

No diagnosis, no treatment, but the urine output overnight was abnormally low. The test of renal function showed elevated BUN and creatinine levels. No cause was found.

He again apologized and said, "I am just dying and that cannot be changed."

The next day, renal function was worse, his respiratory rate was increased, and he was bluish in color, so nasal cannula oxygen was started. Unsuccessful diuretic therapy was begun.

The next day, he was confused and disoriented. His liver function studies had suddenly become elevated. The WBC count was increased, the Hgb fell, the platelets became low, and petechiae were noted.

Blood cultures were all negative, urine culture was also negative.

On the fourth day, he was neurologically unresponsive, subcutaneous bleeding was noted, liver function test results were extremely high, and his breathing had become labored.

Later that afternoon, he peacefully died with his family at the bedside.

An autopsy was requested by his family, but no cause for his deterioration was found. He just had changes compatible with his seventy-seven years of living. But he died, nevertheless.

Some mysteries are never solved, here there was some active process that only the patient could detect. Everyone else remained confused and saddened. No answer again!

There must be something to be found here, but not at that time.

Sepsis is the current terminology for the inflammatory response with organ dysfunction. Other etiologies may also trigger the same general inflammatory response.

In all, there seems to be a grossly similar inflammatory response in all the injuries to the human body.

The response to infection has been a continual source of confusion to all who have ever looked closely at sepsis.

Ignaz Semmelweis noted, without knowing about sepsis, that the course of childbirth fever was not always the same and varied a lot in all women, but it was invariably bad. But the problem is that less than half of all sepsis cases have a positive blood culture, so is infection the only cause of sepsis?

The scholars of the sepsis syndrome over the years of its modern existence have worked diligently to define the syndrome. The differing manifestations of disease seemed to evade a simple definition. Somehow the presentations of the diseases were different.

The best definition of sepsis is a life-threatening organ dysfunction caused by dysregulated host response to disease. In all, this is quite an inclusive definition.

Possibly each condition was truly a unique disease. Multiple syndromes have been cataloged and named due to the observed variable clinical manifestations but in a gross review were not too far from a liberal diagnosis of sepsis.

No specific chemical identifiers of sepsis have been found. Despite the increased amounts of glycocalyx products that enter the circulation during sepsis, this glycocalyx component spill has not shown a specific chemical pattern that would allow diagnosis of sepsis. Even less, this analysis has not been shown to predict sepsis severity. Genomics have also been unable to discriminate to help in clinical diagnosis.

The standard tests of inflammation are performed and then this data must be clinically correlated by the treating physician with each patient's clinical disease in mind.

Algorithms to diagnose sepsis more rapidly and definitely are under development, but problems with ow accuracy interfere. Artificial intelligence has not been able to bridge this algorithm gap.

The current scientific method is to use statistical tools and computer analysis to aid in a more rapid recognition of the benefit of medical interventions have not made the desired differences.

These large statistical studies show that moving rapidly to the administration of right treatments, primarily fluids and antibiotics, does change the outcome in large series with statistical confirmation.

Medical care is improved as a result of these extensive studies, but a single dramatic change has not happened.

Progress is being made in this area. Recently Prokineticin 2 (a new product) has been found to be correlated with sepsis severity and sepsis outcomes. But where will this piece of information fit into the huge puzzle? Much work is underway by many researchers to develop a test or tests that will diagnose sepsis. The ability to clearly define sepsis would be a great forward step.

Individual patient differences are a problem to appreciate and must be quantifiable for computer analysis to be a useful tool in solving these clinical problems.

Treatment programs are bundled (grouped together) as the current clinical approach. These clinically focused treatment plans developed after extensive scientific committee work. The best information must be available in order to be statistically analyzed. The multisource large collections are statistically powered to expose minor differences and prove new answers to help clinical therapy and improve patient outcomes.

The electronic medical record has resulted in hundreds of studies all searching for predictive models. No breakthrough has resulted from this huge amount of work. The electronic medical record has yet to become a productive tool that expands medical research.

The Surviving Sepsis study project is a very extensive review by very knowledgeable investigators of all the available information that has been published. This was a very comprehensive review of all available data by the leaders in Sepsis research.

Today the recommendations made to the clinical services from the sepsis study group are:

1. Do it sooner!
2. Do it faster!
3. Carefully observe the response.
4. Record for statistical processing.
5. Analyze the recorded observations.

Hopefully, these simple clinical observations will lead to further positive supportive measures and modifications.

So, more monitoring is better. More items are included in each new study. The timing of the interventions is now measured and statistically analyzed and recorded in the electronic medical record.

The results have improved outcomes, but adverse outcomes (death) still occur, and the improvements are far too limited. A strong suggestion is made in the editorial section of the *Journal of the American Medical Association* (JAMA) to modify the methods and look to another area to search.

Most disappointingly, no new drugs or treatment modifications or any other interventions have been found in the latest recommendations or in the last fifty years.

Essentially, the problem of sepsis treatment is still unsolved. The answers are here deep within this complex human physiology. Fifty years of searching have not found the answer to sepsis but have defined the human physiology much better.

This scientific stalemate strongly supports a need for another approach. The exquisite detailed biophysiological functions continue to find complex activation programs and whole series of related enzymatic programs. These are true discoveries of human physiologic interactions in the increasing complexity. The ideas that interference in the cytokine series would end that pathologic contribution are being developed. Specific drugs have been designed that effectively stop the individual actions, but when applied to the sepsis syndrome clinically, only a partial benefit is obtained. This is a failure of linear response testing. This existing scientific process continues and publishes volumes of data.

The research efforts also look at the immune system, also an area of focus. Traumatic injury is proven to cause an acquired immunodepression. Associated cellular dysfunction is an integral part of this dysfunction, but this work has yet to develop any positive interventions. Trauma also induces the inflammatory response.

The newest developments seem to portend some good will eventually result. Still another area of fruitless effort. Nothing new here, either!

The various proteins and glycoproteins have been discussed (mostly listed) in the previous chapter and have become the basis of the new explanations and show the vagaries of the active disease process.

In our review, the same injuries result in quite varied responses. The responses are not a single linear reaction (A causes B causes C causes . . .). The explanation of the disease progression process as a single pathway is not adequate to answer all the questions. In essence, complexity is made even more complex.

Because so little progress is being made, a fresh look at sepsis may be in order.

A new mechanism of the inflammatory disease process is proposed.

This new theory expands the areas of focus beyond our current explanations of the status of the inflammatory process. This theory is a speculative explanation and must be considered in the light of creation.

The earlier discussion of the endothelial glycocalyx (EGLX) function is accepted as a basic gross beginning.

When the EGLX is intact, the system functions well and the patient is well.

When the EGLX is injured, a pathologic disease process begins.

This theory presents a different definition of "wellness." This definition states: Damage to the EGLX results in sepsis disease manifestation.

Varied insults injure the EGLX. Each injury can be imagined to be unique in the type and the extent of the injury and the variations in the timing of the injury. When different systems and enzymes are involved without controlling the extent, anything can happen.

These explanations appear to be plausible but cannot be proven to any degree.

The chaos theory best defines the varied unpredictable responses that occur. *The Oxford Dictionary* defines chaos theory as the branch of mathematics that deals with complex systems whose behavior is highly sensitive to slight changes in conditions, so that small alterations can give rise to strikingly great consequences.

Common use of this term chaos generally has a random and inconsistent pattern of responses resulting in great difficulty when describing and understanding the observation,

Chaos allows the classically described and the variations of the same disease to be manifested. This chaos manifestation pattern can be discussed because chaos allows speculations of variable mechanisms and also differences of activation and interactions to be observed.

A simple example clarifies how an injury inducement of the disease can work.

1. When an automobile is driven on a paved road without road damage, a smooth ride is the result.

2. But when the automobile strikes a small pothole, little or no damage results but a bump is noted and no other problems seem to occur and the car proceeds normally.

3. But when the automobile strikes a large pothole, definite damage is done (a flat tire, disrupted steering, or an accident but the exact damage is not predictable). The damage results in "dysfunction" of the car and repairs must be performed.

4. But when the automobile strikes a very deep hole, the entire car can be destroyed, or such damaged parts make the car unworkable. But it can be fixed with difficulty.

5. The hole is so deep the damage is so severe that nothing can be done. The car is obviously totally destroyed. This last example

is relatively equivalent to the onset of sepsis, and the entire organism is destroyed. Descriptions of automobile damage is used because this analogy is a quite familiar. Road damage is a poorly-defined problem, but road damage has a common basis for understanding accidents.

The patterns of injury have not been published or discussed. This series of cartoon illustrations is only the author's attempt to exemplify how injuries can have dissimilar stages and therefore trigger different pathophysiologic reactions.

These cartoons also allow development of the concept of diffuse damages that have widely varied locations and may or may not be related. The concept of variability and intensity of glycocalyx injury caused by the "noxious agent" can be explained by this concept. Randomness of damage to all depths and occurring at random geographic locations and may act to trigger different intensities of inflammatory response. This randomness of injury also presents a basis for consideration of the severity and the inconsistent progression of the sepsis syndrome.

This also supports the chaos discussion presented earlier in the book.

This Table provides the six levels of theoretical injury. This is an illustration-drawing that presents one explanation of the potential degrees of injury and the results.

All these illustrations are a speculative method for classification to rate injury for clarification and recording using this staging system.

This is a sketch compilation of the theoretical patterns of damage to the endothelial glycocalyx. The injury pattern is assumed to be random in location, depth, and area of injury. This is designed to provide a skeletal structure for consideration of severity of injury that may relate to the various manifestations of the inflammatory

Classification of Sepsis Pathology
Staging of Endothelial Glycocalyx Damage

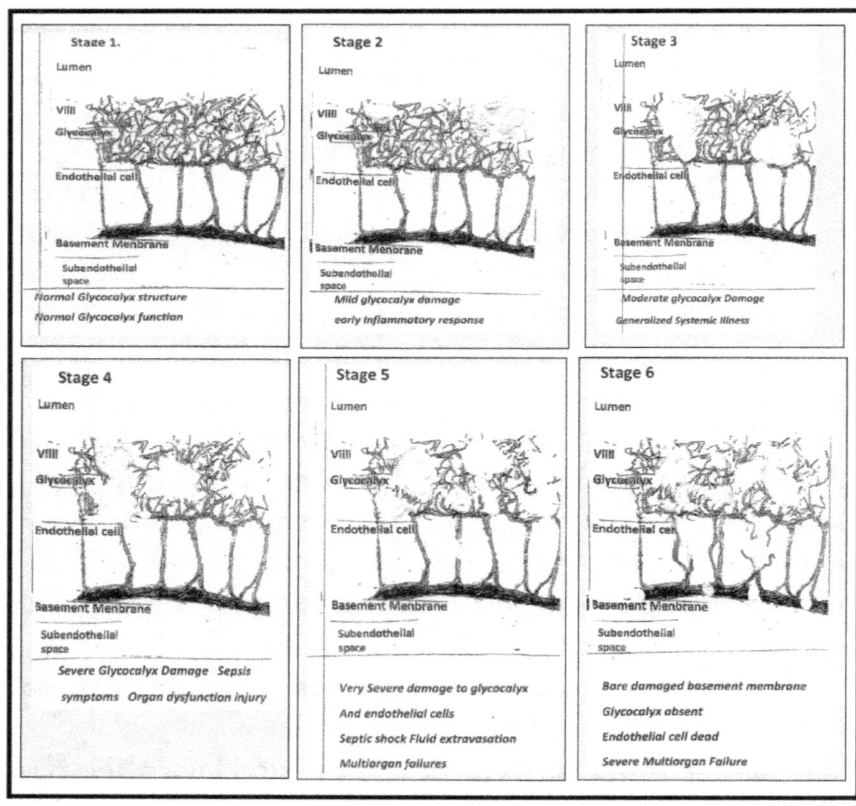

A theoretical pattern of injury can be created based on general knowledge of endothelial glycocalyx anatomic structure.

The clinical observations of presentations of sepsis support this classification.

The injury is presumed to be variable in location and severity. This chart assumes the observed clinical features reflect the most severe manifestation of the sepsis disease.

responses. Stages of involvement can be assigned.

This chart of "anatomic" injury is a new presentation created without any documented scientific support whatsoever. This discussion does supply a theoretical explanation that matches the chaotic pattern seen clinically. Supportive data will surely be found that could reinforce and/or alter the theory to make it more likely to be correct.

One goal of sepsis research committee is to find a defined consensus and definition that all can use and build an algorithm for all to use.

When a classification schedule was attempted, the initial attempts were chaos. What a coincidence! The pattern of inflammatory response is best described by applying the chaos theory. Sepsis is still a very dynamic disease (concept).

When all the damage variables are considered, such as the time of injury, the duration of the injury, the depth of the injury, the size pf the injury, and the varying types of the injury, the number and patterns that can result are many. A dominant distribution pattern can develop or not.

Therefore, observed physiologic patterns appear to suggest that distinctly different diseases are present when that may just be an optional expression of the glycocalyx response.

The statistical method of disease analysis will continue the confusion until more and better ways of classifying data are found and the conclusions are validated by sepsis itself.

These presenting patterns seem to be related to specified damage and random geographical pattern of injury to the EGLX. A case can be made that different proteoglycans are exposed to begin their specifically defined activation process. Whether it is primarily platelet activation, or the coagulation pathway, or the thrombotic pathway, or leukocyte, activation certainly will present its individual reactions.

The inflammatory cascade activation seems to be a random response to an injury to the EGLX layer.

More than one pathophysiologic disease system may originate

from the same area of injury to the glycocalyx. All the affected systems begin their pathological progression in the glycocalyx to create disease. Is there any information currently available? Minimal if any data is available to clarify these concerns.

Many other areas and proteoglycan systems may also be triggered uniformly or sequentially. Inasmuch as the source of the damage persists or recurs, the injury process may continue. The mechanisms of injury have not yet been defined.

The massive area of the glycocalyx suggests that many different areas may be damaged, and that widespread damage is unlikely to be uniform in its inflammatory response. The original concept of inflammatory response to any noxious item occurred very frequently, and the inflammatory activation was quickly followed by local control and then repair. No permanent harm was done, and homeostasis was re-established and maintained.

The observed specifics of the "disease" that are clinically observed are the end-stage manifestations of incited activation of specific proteolytic enzyme systems. This cascade explanation suggests the inflammatory response is a very active and quite variable pattern. The progression and dominance of the initial basic pathologic inflammatory process to the clinical manifestation of the septic disease is not defined. Very little has been shown about the dynamics leading to progression of sepsis.

The clinical sepsis disease pattern may be manifested early or later in the pathological process. Currently there are no specific expected or predicted responses when an inciting incident is noted.

Only the most prominent aspects of sepsis are clinically recognized. Interventions are then appropriately applied. Since only supportive measures are available, the criteria for the treatment of specific recognized problems by the interventions for that problem are activated.

The supportive responses that do not result in positive clinical interventions are generally not published in the literature. These absent data points compromise our thought process because we only see half or less of the potentially helpful information. (The puzzle piece did not fit—a negative answer, but no one knows about it.)

The pattern of statistical analysis currently in vogue is to acquire a large and substantial number of cases and drill down on that data searching for consistent answers. This technique needs specific, easily definable and measurable markers and the classifier must then omit subtle changes and findings to assure an adequate number of cases for analysis.

This investigative technique seems to be nearly incompatible with the chaotic disease of sepsis. Areas of prior study are reviewed but new areas of study are limited and do not fit well with the greater statistical analysis methods. To make the techniques work, a considerable amount of data that does not meet criteria is simply ignored or the presentations are modified.

This is extremely tough research and technically problematic with extremely difficult data analysis. Progress is slow or nonexistent. Despite that, everyone is diligently working to find a solution to the major human killer that is sepsis, but our current progress is limited. Hundreds of studies have been performed and more are in process primarily doing similar analytic activities.

The new description of the inflammatory cascade activated within the glycocalyx and endothelial cells presents a new and different look at the refractory problem of sepsis.

The lack of linkages and varied sites and patterns of injury are so poorly defined that the best efforts frequently do not find answers. The best explanation of the multiple patterns and presentation results is **chaos**.

Today, chaos may be the best explanation of the variable presentations of sepsis.

Are they looking in the right place, or just where the light is best?

CHAPTER EIGHT

Look Out Sepsis!
Here comes The Norberg Solution!

The life of rules and games is such a large part of society; mostly they come with limited consideration of their value. But certainly, these rules are to be followed.

Social resistance to change slows the introduction of even the most beneficial changes. With this background of delayed social acceptance, the technical aspects of discovery are completed early, but then are followed by a slow introduction and eventually gain acceptance and full incorporation into our lives.

TNS (The Norberg Solution), a product that will eventually be found to treat sepsis, was a dead issue so many times in its development. However, as each total obstruction was encountered, and progress stopped, the situation changed and each obstacle was overcome. There was something extra (the clinical force) that helped get TNS through and around all the deadly obstructions and barricades over the long period of time. TNS developed following a course that was previously not even considered because of rules. TNS magically found and made its way through the maze. More details later.

Our least known systemic organ, EGLX, can be the site of change, so we can expect a controversial introduction as change is deadly!

The last and best definition of sepsis was presented in the last Surviving Sepsis Conference Report 2020. Sepsis is **a life-threatening organ dysfunction due to a dysregulated host response from an infection.**

Sepsis is a whole-body systemic inflammatory response that is uncontrolled. The common presenting signs are fever, increased heart rate, increased rate of breathing, confusion, and hypotension. The localized site of infection may provide more signs and support the diagnosis. Septic shock is a subset in which profound circulatory, cellular, and metabolic abnormalities carry a greater risk of mortality.

Clinically, the patient is sick. Fever may or may not be present, pulse is increased, and blood pressure and perfusion may be diminished. Delirium shows some central nervous system dysfunction. Usually, a specific organ shows dysfunction, e.g., urinary tract, breathing difficulty, or abdominal pain or distention rapidly help in the diagnosis and formulation of a program of prompt treatment.

The prognosis in sepsis treatment has been stifled. And the mortality rate remains unchanged.

The current Critical Care medical response recommended is a "bundled approach." Essentially, this can be summarized as, "Do it all! And now!"

This is the consensus report of the Surviving Sepsis Conference Report of 2020.

The problem of circulatory failure is fluid loss into the tissues. This is tackled by addressing copious amounts of crystalloid fluids that rapidly leave the vascular space and cause "third spacing" or massive edema and swelling of the entire body, including the face. Multiorgan failure follows and may lead to death. Even the timing and use of vasopressors to manage the shock is not a clear recommendation today.

Increased white blood cell counts are present and platelet counts are low. Bruising may be present or petechiae or seen and when obtained abnormalities of the coagulation system are found.

Metabolic dysfunction is shown by systemic lactic acidosis along with electrolyte abnormalities that are often present at the onset of the illness.

Central nervous system presentation is an altered level of consciousness, but the patient is usually responsive (delirious) and this is not usually considered a severe part of the problem. Typical management is observation and sedation.

Patients who have recovered from sepsis are now being assessed, and their cognitive function is a more important aspect than previously thought. Now, post-ICU rehabilitative programming is becoming a component of Intensive Care Unit patient care. Recovery following sepsis is far more complicated than previously thought.

The sepsis pattern, while individually variably expressed, has a general consistency that requires the bedside clinician to observe changes in presentation and the changing pathophysiology in response to the active medical interventions. This skill is difficult and cannot be acquired from a book or a lecture, which makes it much more difficult to apply medical interventions.

The most obvious problem is shock, and previously the first intervention was to treat the third spacing. This aggressive medical treatment resulted in severe edema to the point of distortion. Often the patient's appearance was changed so severely that it made their mothers cry.

Along with the fluid overload, ARDS made breathing difficult. The impression that the fluid treatment was drowning the patient was hard to avoid. The change in the patient's appearance was the result of the aggressive fluid treatment of the shock.

This persistent circulatory failure caused by the recurrent hypovolemia and vasodilation was compounded by fluid loss into the extracellular space.

It is clear that the massive amounts of crystalloid fluids that were required to keep up the circulating volume that the patient needed had to be retained within the vascular system. The circulatory failure caused urinary output to be low, was treated with diuretics, hopefully to increase urinary output and decrease the edema. The diuretics generally failed to accomplish the desired goal of fluid decrease with increased urinary output.

Regarding the third spacing problem recorded in the multiple studies, the explanation suggested was that "the pores in the basement membrane" were equal to 66 daltons in size, which is the same as the albumin molecule. The solution to the leakage problem was obvious; using a molecule larger than the pore size (the hole) was needed. This larger molecule would stay in circulation and prevent fluid loss into the subcutaneous tissue, as explained by the Starling Principle.

"A larger molecule would be needed to stop the leak." Such a simple answer and a very dim light came on.

Therefore, a large molecule was developed, a poly starch product that stayed within the circulation longer but had problems with worsening kidney function and severe itching for the remaining life of the saved patient. This polystarch product is now rarely used.

Large molecules of varied poly starches were created and used to replace albumin. These clinical studies found problems with renal failure, and in some cases permanent urticaria. The conclusion was that poly starches were not an answer to third spacing. The result is now crystalloids are the primary preferred fluids of today. Poly starches still have proponents that advocate their use, but only cautiously and in limited circumstances. In current medical therapy, starches are not part of routine treatments. Natural albumin had little if any advantage over crystalloids.

From the clinical bedside, this third spacing was at best a very vexing problem. The logical answer was to use serum albumin for volume replacement. In multiple studies of volume replacement, the results using albumin were only slightly better than crystalloid fluids results. The entire Critical Care specialty uses albumin frequently but is not satisfied that it is adequate.

The return to crystalloids was the modern clinical approach. In the June 2022 issue of the *New England Journal of Medicine,* a series of different crystalloid fluids and administration rates and volumes were studied. No significant differences in outcomes could be measured and confirmed. "Crystalloids are the best fluids at present."

The search continued, and all products available that were known to be safe and used often were considered.

While albumin had some minimal benefits, augmentation of the albumin molecule size should make it more effective. A new theory was conceived by the author. Albumin in vivo had water molecules passively attached, which could be replaced with amino acid molecules.

A logical combination was to put albumin and hydrolyzed amino acids together. Both products were composed of amino acids as the base products, but the albumin structure was formed from the amino acids into a specifically-sequenced long chain that is complexly folded. This molecular structure is the known pattern in nature.

Could amino acids alter the albumin presentation? The amino acids could be presented as individual molecules to the albumin molecule and develop different forms of bonding and structure.

This raised the consideration that the amino acids could increase the bulk of the albumin to a size too large to escape the vascular space. This new product would become an effective volume expansion product.

Neither albumin nor the hydrolyzed amino acid solutions products have any intrinsic physiological actions or metabolic contributions. Both had been used in medical treatments for more than fifty years. The products have also been used in treatment for more than fifty years without complications. The inert quality of both products made this combination seem a likely possibility.

To confirm that this combination did not create a problem when compounded together, a review of the basic chemical property was performed. Where and how do these amino acids create the changes? Is it by passive bonding or are these amino acids incorporated into the long stream of the albumin?

To obtain some answers to determine whether the albumin would be different, a study was requested of a university school of pharmacy to perform a study to define the physical characteristics of this new compound.

The physical characteristic analysis showed that the potential worrisome condition, that of agglutination (clumping), did not occur. The combination albumin and amino acid solution did not gel or show a change in viscosity when compared to natural albumin. Further studies focusing on the potential problem of polymerization were negative; polymerization was not present.

Continuing testing continued evaluating the consistency of molecular size "variability" compared to the native albumin size variability. The constancy of the size variability was similar. A polydispersity analysis showed no significant differences compared to albumin alone.

Albumin is a chemically inactive product and has no effect on any other system. Amino acids also have no intrinsic chemical activity. Both products have a history of familiarity with more than fifty years of clinical application.

The resultant detailed chemical analysis report was so very encouraging that this new albumin product met all the desired parameters, although size was minimally increased.

The desired primary goal, to create an increased volume albumin molecule, this result had truly occurred. This larger size was measured and determined to be a 17 percent increase in size. Statistically, this size was a significant difference (meaning the measurements were correct).

Physiologically, the size increase of 17 percent was initially considered to be too small to have any clinical effect. Only clinical testing could determine the significance of that change. TNS was the first product compounded, and only clinical testing over time could tell how beneficial this change would be. Testing would be more complicated, as albumin is a species-specific product. Animal studies will not suffice.

This combination product was shown to be a product that initially appeared to meet the requirements to be an acceptable volume replacement product.

This new product would need a name. Historically, fluids have been named after their inventor. This product was named after the inventor, William Norberg MD. This is now **The Norberg Solution** and the abbreviated name became **TNS.** TNS is now a reality and ready to go.

The introduction of TNS to the world was met with: **Not so quick, there**!

There are a lot of procedural hurdles and established protocols along with new and old rules and requirements to comply with before TNS could go forward.

Federal Drug Administration of the USA (FDA) classifications presented total obstructions. The cost was prohibitive and the rules complex. FDA compliance could not be achieved. This approach required more support, and that was not available. Initial new drug application fees were millions of dollars.

Albumin was classified as a **biologic product** and was assigned and controlled by the Biological Division of the FDA and could not be combined with any other products of any type.

The amino acid solution was defined as a **pharmaceutical product** and assigned to and controlled by the Pharmaceutical Division of the FDA.

Longstanding FDA regulations prohibited the mixing of these two products. Biologics and pharmaceutical products had rules designed to create completely independent FDA divisions. There was no option for crossing that established bureaucratic line!

That was the end of TNS!

"Biologicals and pharmaceuticals shall never meet or mix." USA FDA

All stops here! This can't be done!

The new, larger albumin project ended at this point. Well, this really was a stop and wait point. Waiting was begun with faith that something good would eventually happen.

In 2005, the problem of the newly-invented insulin pumps and safe insulin administration forced the FDA to address and fix the artificial barrier designation problem. The vast separations within the FDA could no longer exist; the boundaries had been breached. New regulations were provided.

A new category of COMPOUNDED MEDICAL PRODUCTS has been set up. This new albumin and amino acid combination easily met the combination product definition.

Getting over the first barrier occurred early and was solved by spontaneous evolution of the FDA system.

This newly-discovered albumin amino acid mixture (TNS) was now an accorded combination product.

How many more obstructions would be found?

As the solution to the third spacing problem in sepsis, this new albumin product, TNS, should solve the problem.

It was believed that the whole world would soon arrive at the door and fully adopt this new treatment!

Hallelujah!

Not so at all!

Once again, the old adage failed to deliver! A better mouse trap will not bring the world to your door. One more time with the same result.

Big Pharma had a clear and tepid response, "You do all the hard work of development, take all the risk, and then we will buy the product from you. But no money now!"

All the drug manufacturers seemed to have read the same book and gave the same answer: No money now!

Okay, the Government has lots of funding and is interested in new products. The National Institute of Health (NIH) and other government agencies had extremely strict requirements. A lot of time and money went into learning about these government programs and learning the rules of the road. Their strict requirements could not be met.

TNS was developed by a lone entrepreneur associated with an academic university, but without access to the formal academic financial structure. TNS did not originate from a formal research laboratory. No funding from here.

The TNS product therefore did not meet the official requirements of NIH or any other government programs. No financial support was available from any U.S. government programs.

Angel investors are reputed to be a wonderful basic form of support.

The first rule of angel investing is that the inventor must get all the money possible from your relatives as the first step, and then the "Angels" will rescue you all. Their motto seems to be that if your own mother will not support you, why would we?

Additionally, the angel investors asked how much money was needed? And for how long? And more critically, when the financial return would start. Since the timing and funding were unknown, the result was **no support**.

It was not surprising that these terribly negative experiences resulted in a hold on TNS development.

Time passed, and there seemed to be no way to get TNS into patient care. None of the people wanted to take even a minimal risk to save lives! One pharma representative explicitly said, "We are busy, and we are making money, why take any risk that may not pay off?"

Only in a legitimate and ethical way could the TNS development go ahead. No patient treatment could be done. All the ethical legal criteria were reviewed, and no options seemed possible.

Attempts to find and recruit other critical care physicians and intensive care programs to work in concert were unsuccessful. The physicians initially clearly expressed interest and developed an understanding of TNS, supplying strong intellectual support of the concept. But beyond verbal support, no adopters resulted from these efforts.

The search for other researchers and sites identified by the scientists working on sepsis all supplied moral support. Thes public exposures did not bear fruit. The whole field of medicine and the pharmacological industry nodded interestingly and gave the"HMMMMM".

Presentations to the scientific committees of the Society of Critical Care Medicine (SCCM) listened attentively, but nothing more. A booth at the annual congress of the SCCM drew interesting comments and helpful suggestions, but nothing more.

Direct application to the FDA for a new drug application was made. This was a very time-consuming effort for a single researcher with full-time critical care practice. Discounted licensing fees were offered by the FDA to small entity companies. The fee was discounted to a mere $1,119,000 and came with the government's reassurance of further discounted fees in the future. These excessive licensing costs precluded pursuing the FDA's new drug application track.

During this time, this personally funded research continued. More was learned about human physiology and the dysfunction associated with sepsis. Medical supportive measures were developed and refined and applied, but not TNS. Direct patient care improved, but still no cure for sepsis.

For TNS, no progress or even activity was happening. The first bottle of TNS just sat and gathered dust.

TNS was ready but there was nowhere to go. This appeared to be the classic dead end. All known legitimate avenues had been explored.

But, if you believe and wait, something good will happen!

The government did it! The government did it!

A new federal law, the Drug and Safety Act of 2013, was passed in response to a series of fungal infections in commercially compounded pharmaceutical products. New regulations were revised to supply safe compounded products. A section of this bill authorized physicians to prescribe and for pharmacists to fulfil the product to be used in the physician's direct treatment of his patients.

In 2018, a new guidance document was released by the FDA titled "Mixing, Diluting, or Repackaging Biological Products Outside the Scope of an Approved Biologics License Application Guidance for Industry."

This regulatory clarification allowed patient treatment with TNS under direct physician prescription when the TNS was prepared by a pharmacist for the treatment of a specific medical problem in a patient of the physician.

The compounding of medicines and potions is an ancient art and continues to be an essential aspect of modern medicine. The guidance related primarily to the preservation of the sterility and the preservation of the products throughout the packaging, storage, and transfer of the compounded products. No prior guidance had ever been provided, but the rules were easily adopted, as they were the same rules used daily in most hospital pharmacies.

This guidance publication eliminated the confusion that developed in pharmacies when TNS compounding was requested.

A review of that guidance vehicle would resolve the concerns of the pharmacists and their lawyers and administrators. The pharmaceutical industry would address and solve this problem.

TNS clearly meets the known safe product for use criteria. The mixing procedure in the sterile suites of the hospital pharmacy or compounding pharmacy meets the production criteria. The preservation, transport, and storage remain somewhat vague, but the compounded product should be used directly and definitely within the labeled shelf lifetime of human serum albumin shown on the packaging. These shelf-life criteria are established by the compounding agency who maintains responsible for the safety of the product.

TNS consists of two of medicine's safest products. Human serum albumin has no allergic risk, no incompatibility, is chemically inactive, and is the major protein in the human body. The physical characteristic is like albumin in viscosity in freedom from agglutination and polymerization, with presumed long-time stability at room temperature. The hydrolyzed amino acid solution is the building blocks of all proteins. This product has been used regularly in treatment programs for more than fifty years with no adverse effects.

This FDA ruling change opened the door to patient treatment with TNS within the USA. The regulating agencies across the world generally have and/or follow the USA FDA patterns of regulations.

A development plan for TNS was carefully and slowly developed to avoid any violations of hospital rules, regulations, and by-laws. The restrictive intuitional research regulation by individual hospital Investigational Research Boards provides ethics guidance for patient-related scientific research. These rules were reviewed and conscientiously accepted. Full compliance was assured with all ethics guidance and patient research regulations. All clinical actions were in full compliance with everything found. Patient consent was not needed, as the hospital administration defined this as a treatment activity that was approved by the patient care authorizations completed on hospital admission. HIPPA rules were in full compliance and were carefully and completely adhered to.

There seemed to be no further regulatory or other legal barriers to TNS use in patient care.

So many years of frustration and disappointment had been endured, but now all that was in the past. TNS could be used to save patients' lives.

Halleluiah!

Here it goes!

CHAPTER NINE

TNS Takes on Sepsis and Wins!

This chapter includes more direct medical terminology that is used to describe the medical activities and patient responses better and more exactly. The medical terminology and patterns relate back directly to patient medical care records.

Here are the true-life stories of patients who were treated with TNS. Their outcomes demonstrate the beneficial effect of TNS. Direct patient therapy with TNS changed the patient's status in a miraculous way: all patients survived and benefited.

This description is provided to show how this miracle came to be. This new miracle is presented to all the world. The number of patients treated is limited, but the physiologic changes are so unique and dramatic that these changes cannot be ignored.

These changes are easily recognized by the treating physicians and their nursing colleagues. Because the recovery pattern of the TNS-treated people is so remarkably different than everyone's expected experiences, these medical breakthroughs are easily recognized.

The scientific observation method works!

The double blinded pattern of scientific study is replaced by the case report method for TNS. Comparison data for the recognition of changes depends on the clinician's own personal experience.

Only a very few clinical cases are presented, but the variation from the "standard expected case outcome" opens our minds to a consideration of **a new paradigm in medical treatment**. This feat required direct patient care experience.

Only after all these years of tedious work to ensure complete compliance on all accounts was completed could TNS administration for patient treatment be used. Everything had to be correct and in place. There could be no room for error. These treatments did all meet ethical standards.

The cases presented are all known patients, but their medical records and the patients are not identified as required by HIPAA (A USA Program).

TNS was accepted for use for medical treatment when the proper clinical application was needed. TNS will be clinically determined to be the right medical therapy for that moment in the patient's life. End-stage desperate applications are unlikely to benefit or change outcomes and will likely only confound legitimate medical conclusions. This exception is a reasonable presumption today, but does anyone truly know why it should be?

Remarkably, TNS can be used as an additional therapy without modification of the existing medical treatment. Nothing must be changed, limited, or stopped when TNS is added to the treatment program. Allergy and immune reactions are not problems.

TNS meets the MAGIC BULLET CRITRIA:

TNS has no interaction with existing treatments.

TNS has no allergic or immunologic risk.

TNS uncomplicated production is universally available in all major hospitals.

TNS components are universally available.

TNS is a cheap medical product to provide.

Miracle Case Number One

One late afternoon, a baby was accepted into the Pediatric Intensive Care Unit (PICU) because of her mother's demand that something be done about the baby's severe fluid overload. The patient had Total Parenteral Nutrition (TPN) with intravenous fluids prescribed and was retaining fluids.

She was admitted for the treatment of severe dehydration due to recurrent partial bowel obstruction. She had been known to this hospital since infancy when she was treated for Hirschsprung's Disease and received an ileostomy as the initial therapy. Recurrent ileal prolapse caused repeated episodes of bowel obstruction, causing malnutrition.

The ileal prolapse had recurred and the infant was very dehydrated. The baby was rehydrated without problems initially. To address the malnutrition, she was started on a TPN program. She developed a complication with severe third spacing of fluids coupled with borderline hypoperfusion.

Diuretic therapy had been prescribed to control the edema, but it was ineffective in treating the third spacing. The edema was steadily worsening to severe generalized body edema with ascites (fluid within the abdomen). The swelling of her face was so severe that her eyes were almost swollen shut. She barely resembled herself.

The medical history, examination, and the medical record showed the diagnosis of Hirschsprung's disease promptly recognized in the neonatal period. The standard treatment was an ileostomy.

Home care was difficult due to recurrent episodes of extensive small bowel prolapse. Each episode caused bowel obstruction and complete interruption of feeding resulting in malnutrition. She was unable to follow the expected growth chart for normal babies.

At PICU admission, she was noted to be massively fluid overloaded. Anasarca was severe; she was barely able to open her eyes to see. She was also very miserable, and in severe distress. The usual measures to calm her failed and she persisted with a weak cry and fussiness. Her medical treatments had failed and now the third spacing created a critical situation.

Her mother was fully aware of the severity of the problem and extremely anxious and crying while her husband was trying to comfort her. A full discussion of the current medical situation was provided to both parents.

The available treatment options included hemodialysis or hemo-ultra-filtration to remove fluids rapidly. Both of these are invasive procedures that require central vessel cannulation of veins and arteries under anesthesia. These procedures are difficult in small infants. These are complex medical procedures but are standardly applied therapies within the PICU.

During the discussion of possible dialysis and their difficulty, her mother asked if there was something else that could be done.

The case had been reviewed and there were no contraindications to TNS treatment. TNS failure would only cause a short delay before starting hemo-ultra filtration procedures and beginning of treatments. It did not appear the use of TNS provided significant risk. TNS treatment was offered, and the family accepted.

She was to be the first patient ever to receive TNS. A historic but not in any way dramatic episode.

Therefore, TNS was administered to improve blood pressure control and prevent further fluid overload.

The TNS was administered judiciously, as this was our first administration. She showed steady improvement when the TNS was started. Urine output increased subjectively; her perfusion improved. The whole infusion was accomplished without any clinical instability. A second dose was administered after twelve hours for continued circulatory volume support and fluid stabilization.

The next morning, at the onset of the day shift nursing report, the nursing notes stated "resting comfortability, no edema." The edema had resolved rapidly overnight! The periorbital edema was gone, the ascites was gone. The baby appeared happy and well.

All the fluid problems present on PICU admission had completely resolved!

A negative fluid loss of 1.9 kg was recorded. Laboratory studies were all normal.

Nothing like this fluid mobilization had ever been seen! All this dramatic change happened without any instability. The baby appeared "happy and well!" How could that happen?

Routine support measures, including the TPN, were continued until the presenting problem of partial bowel obstruction due to small bowel prolapse was corrected. The third spacing never recurred. No additional TNS was given.

The child improved rapidly and was discharged home.

This was the first MIRACLE clinical recovery.

The many years of direct PICU patient care had taught me what the expected patterns should be and in what timeframe. This patient's response met none of the predicted outcomes.

This case did not follow the rules. It was unlike anything that had ever happened before.

This rapid resolution of edema in a patient with the problem of active third spacing of fluid resistant to diuretic treatment was a new phenomenon. This had never occurred in such a short time frame or with this degree of severity.

This rapid correction of third spacing during fluid management reinforced the original premise that "increased albumin molecular size" had facilitated the extracellular fluid mobilization.

This was interpreted as a therapeutic breakthrough in fluid management. This was the first case ever!

THIS IS A NEW MEDICAL PHENOMONEN THAT HAS NEVER BEEN SEEN BEFORE!

Miracle Case Number Two

The second patient to ever receive TNS was a male infant initially admitted to the PICU for treatment of intussusception causing a bowel obstruction. On presentation he was quite ill and had been vomiting for two days. The examination was positive for dehydration and absent bowel sounds, an enlarged abdomen, and dehydration.

His initial therapy was customary; early institution of broad-spectrum antibiotics and bolus crystalloid fluids to treat dehydration. A therapeutic barium enema was the next step. It was performed; but this therapeutic maneuver did not relieve the intussusception.

Continued fluid resuscitation with normal saline boluses corrected his dehydration, and he was ready for surgery.

Upon opening the abdomen, a very dilated small bowel was noted and the intusseption was isolated. The small bowel had been caught and brought into the large bowel, and the normal action of peristalsis pulled the ileum into the colon, stopping only when it as far as it would go. The small bowel was gently pulled from the large bowel, relieving the obstruction. A period of supported observation of the status of this bowel segment was disappointing; the circulation did not return and the bowel appeared to be dead. Resection of the dead distal ileum and cecum was necessary. Direct anastomosis was performed. The baby tolerated this surgery and was returned to his bed in the PICU.

Multiple boluses of saline were given to keep adequate blood pressure and ensure urinary output throughout the night.

The following day, multiple concerns about bowel viability and possible bowel leakage provided a surgical indication for a second look procedure in the extremely ill infant.

At surgery, the intestinal anastomosis was intact and the remaining bowel was viable, but a severe inflammatory and peritoneal reaction was clear. Cultures were taken, the peritoneal space was irrigated with warmed normal saline, and the abdomen closed primarily.

Upon return to the PICU, an additional saline bolus was administered. More fluids were needed through the night. Severe progressive edema developed, and scrotal fluid increased in volume. Broad-spectrum antibiotics were continued. His clinical course indicated sepsis disease. The blood and peritoneal cultures were pending.

During rounds the following morning, the patient's father was very agitated. He asked many questions about fluids and was especially worried about the massive scrotal swelling that had by that time increased to about 2/3 of the size of the infant's head. His penis was buried deep in the scrotal swelling and could be found only by following the indwelling Foley catheter entering this massive translucent mass. His abdomen was also massively enlarged. Facial disfigurement from severe edema caused his appearance to be gross. It was a terrible scene, and all the family members were afraid.

The usual explanations of fluid communication with the abdomen were given and the medical rationale for the large amounts of fluid the baby had received was presented. His father pointedly asked what was to be done about this massive fluid overload.

This baby's time in the hospital overlapped the first case of TNS given, and the father was aware that another child had been given something that stopped and fixed the fluid overload.

Naturally, he asked that the same treatment be given to his son. Although the initial TNS application plan was to avoid critically ill patients early in the TNS experience, this critically ill infant was not responding to our treatments and was looking poorly.

He appeared likely to die. TNS could be an appropriate rescue treatment. (This was clearly an exception to the original plan to avoid critically ill patients who could die. Withholding treatment did not seem to be a right thing to do!)

TNS was administered slowly and safely without changes in his vital signs or general status. The TNS treatment was repeated in twelve hours. Maintenance fluids were kept at very minimal rates.

The patient promptly became afebrile, and the fluid overload very rapidly resolved. The scrotal size returned to normal promptly in twenty-four hours. The patient showed resolution of edema and ascites within the first forty-eight hours.

This patient again had an unbelievable reversal of his downhill course. He had been following a pathway to death.

His appearance and his clinical status improved more rapidly than expected.

The patient had a surprisingly rapid and unremarkable recovery.

He had been considered highly likely to die from sepsis with multiorgan failure. His treatment and survival were considered remarkable successes.

Nothing like this had been seen before in this PICU.

His family was incredibly pleased with his recovery. They did not understand or recognize their baby's miraculous recovery. A live happy baby was what they had expected.

In summary, TNS treatment changed the whole situation and circulatory volume was stabilized. Urinary output increased and the edema began to resolve in the first twenty-four hours. The fever resolved and the recovery from this very critical state was more rapid than ever before seen.

Every good thing that could happen, did happen for this baby.

Conclusion: Patient had volume restoration and diuresis of excessive fluids without problems leading to a much better recovery course. The inflammatory aspect of his sepsis disease was very mild.

TNS significantly altered his recovery course in a manner not previously seen.

Miracle Case Number Three

The patient was a 10-year-old female with known multiple abdominal cystic hygromas and lymphangiectasis. This diagnosis was made initially at age six during a prolonged course of treatments for pleural effusions (empyema) and persistent peritoneal drainage due to the lymphangioma. She has done well during the four-year interval.

She presented acutely with abdominal pain and large right pleural effusion with moderate respiratory distress. O^2 saturation was 90 percent.

Her treatment consisted of broad-spectrum antibiotics at once, and she underwent a Visually Assisted Thoroscopy (VATS) to drain a large pleural empyema and placement of a chest tube.

She was intubated for surgery and full ventilatory support was continued postoperatively.

A CT scan assessed the abdominal disease and showed a large left pleural effusion and ascites. A left chest tube placed and the effusion drained.

She slowly improved with decreasing ventilator setting and decreased O^2 need. Chest tube losses were monitored and replaced intermittently.

TPN was started and the pleural and peritoneal fluid losses were added to the TPN maintenance fluids.

Over the next week, the patient gradually developed generalized edema despite diuretic treatment with an adequate clinical response and full nutritional support. The result was mild but progressive anasarca.

Her mother had seen the rapid fluid mobilization that happened to the other two children. This was the result of PICU waiting room conversations with the other two families. She specifically requested the use of TNS to manage her daughter's systemic fluid overload.

TNS at 15 ml (about 0.51 oz)/kg was administered for total of six doses over two days with continuing diuretic treatment.

The fluid mobilized, chest tube and peritoneal drainage decreased markedly, and the patient could be extubated.

A repeat CT of the abdomen showed resolution of the pleural effusions and an intraabdominal abscess. The abscess was percutaneously drained and the cultures were negative.

Her remaining hospital course was uneventful. She had resolution of the multiple drainage sites over the next five days and was discharged three days after the drains were removed. (This hospital course was short compared to the prior hospitalization.)

This was a complex case with the congenital disease lymphangiomatosis with pleural infection and peritonitis. Her condition improved much beyond mere fluid mobilization. The fluid leakage was promptly resolved and the peritonitis and abdominal abscess cleared rapidly. Again, the rapidity of the fluid mobilization was such a remarkable change in this difficult post-surgical case complicated by documented sepsis. The initial illness course was complicated by severe third spacing of fluids. The patient never had the infusion of albumin provided for correction of hypoalbuminemia.

TNS caused fluid mobilization and decreased the fever and the infections resolved with antibiotic treatment. This had not happened during her first presentation years before. (She provided some information to act as her own control.)

Her mother knew her daughter had benefited from TNS. She emphasized that this hospitalization was so different than the previous hospitalization. Sher credited TNS for the correction of the fluid leakages, and TNS also promoted rapid recovery.

TNS modified fluid dynamics and diminished the inflammatory response like the previous patient.

Miracle Case Number Four

This Patient was a 17-year-old male who had an undefined myopathy. He had a chronic tracheostomy and used his ventilator only at night. He was able to walk independently and performed activities of daily living with only minimal assistance.

He complained of abdominal pain and showed increased weakness for several days, and this problem worsened to progressive abdominal distention and intractable vomiting. After three days of these symptoms, his family took him to the emergency department.

On admission he was extremely ill.

Admission vital signs: Pulse 145, Respirations 14, Blood pressure 108/84.

He was lethargic but oriented when aroused. Extremities were cool to the mid-thigh and capillary filling was delayed at five seconds.

Physical examination: The mucus membranes were dry, and a well healed tracheostomy site with a tracheostomy tube was in place. The respiratory and cardiac examinations were normal. The abdomen was very distended and with absent bowel sounds. Rebound tenderness and guarding was present.

His workup: Abdominal X-ray showed free air in the peritoneal space. The hemoglobin was elevated, the white cell count was high, and electrolytes were in the acceptable range. Protime was twenty-five seconds INR was 2.4 Partial Thromboplastin Time was fifty-five seconds D-Dimer was 2500. An initial fluid bolus of 2500 ml (about 84.54 oz) of normal saline was followed by maintenance IVF at 110 ml (about 3.72 oz)/hour. Intravenous antibiotics (piperacillin tazobactam and clindamycin) were immediately started.

He was brought to surgery. During the anesthesia induction, a disastrous complication happened; he vomited copiously and aspirated gastric contents. The tracheostomy tube was removed, and a cuffed endotracheal tube placed without difficulty. Gastric contents were aspirated from the endotracheal tube. Dopamine was started at ten micrograms per kg/minute via a central line. The situation was controlled, and the operation continued.

The operative findings were pneumatosis intestinalis and bowel distention due to obstructive bands. When the obstruction was relieved, the bowel distention resolved, and the bowel gradually changed from a dusky gray to a pink color. This bowel was deemed viable. The peritoneal space was cultured and then copiously irrigated with normal saline and drains were placed. The surgical incision was closed primarily.

On PICU admission: Vital signs were normal and perfusion appeared adequate with prompt capillary fill. IVF was set at 110 ml (about 3.72 oz)/hour. Dopamine was continued at ten micrograms / kg/minute.

Over the next three hours, the blood pressure decreased slightly, and the pulse increased.

Because of the shock and severe sepsis and known ischemic bowel injury that caused active peritonitis, now combined with an aspiration pulmonary injury, a very difficult post-operative course was anticipated.

A severe septic response with all the complications of sepsis rapidly evolved. The large amounts of crystalloid needed would result in severe respiratory compromise. Third spacing would also occur. Ascites and third spacing would be major problems. Severe pulmonary insufficiency was predictable.

The post-operative care plan was to maintain supportive ventilatory care with O2 as needed, and positioning and suctioning every two hours. Analgesia and sedation as needed. Continuation of antibiotics and other respiratory support measures as needed.

Fluid therapy was an initial infusion of TNS 1000 ml and standard maintenance fluids at 100 ml/hour. TNS 1000 ml would be given every twelve hours and whenever volume was needed.

A total of four doses (4000ml (about 67.63 oz)) each of TNS were administered.

The post-operative course was remarkably different than all his treating physicians had predicted. No pulmonary edema or aspiration pneumonia occurred despite the documented pulmonary aspiration that occurred in surgery.

Five species of klebsiella grew from the peritoneal cultures, thus confirming the diagnosis of sepsis and septic shock. Appropriate antibiotic coverage was continued. Np abscess or peritonitis manifested.

The problems with fluid overload did not occur. Urine output was maintained, electrolytes were unchanged, Ileus resolved rapidly. Recovery was rapid and surprisingly uneventful.

The TNS seems to have provided circulating volume stability, which in turn eliminated the need for crystalloid infusions. With limited fluids, the problems of hyperchloremic acidosis and acute kidney injury appeared to have been avoided. The expected inflammatory response to this severe infection did not occur. No febrile response was ever-present.

The use of the TNS in addition to all other standard sepsis management interventions resulted in an unanticipated benign recovery course. The severe inflammatory responses did not occur and ARDS did not develop, nor did aspiration pneumonia.

Miracle Case Number Five

A twenty-three-year-old male had a complex chromosomal deletion of the long arm of thirteen. His imperforate anus was treated with colostomy and left with a mucus fistula. No further surgical repairs were ever done.

His syndrome also had severe developmental delay and included a generalized seizure disorder.

He had been repeatedly hospitalized for recurrent aspiration pneumonia and had type 1 diabetes mellitus controlled with insulin.

His most recent hospitalization for respiratory failure had resulted in the institution of home ventilator support via a tracheostomy, and his pulmonary status improved dramatically with these interventions.

He suddenly became ill and acutely presented to the emergency department with septic shock. The cause was a urinary tract infection. He responded to IV fluid boluses and urinary tract drainage and antibiotic therapy.

He stabilized on this regimen treating his septic shock. The hospital course was difficult due to a poorly defined ileus and eventually was treated with persistent ileus requiring total parenteral nutrition (TPN).

His type 1 diabetes mellitus was managed with a glucose and Insulin infusion.

His respiratory system was not a problem. He was maintained on his home ventilator at the same settings.

During this hospital course, he had developed lethargy, tachycardia of 165, BP 99/45, capillary fill greater than five seconds, and cold extremities to midthigh. Laboratory studies were normal except for a serum albumin of 1.4 grams percent.

The clinical diagnosis was low cardiac output due to hypovolemia caused by third spacing of fluids. He received 600 TNS for the correction of hypovolemia. The heart rate decreased to 120, BP increased to 100/65, and perfusion improved with warm feet and improved peripheral capillary fill (less than three seconds). He became more alert and responsive, and the edema of his legs and feet decreased over the next day.

The serum albumin increased from 1.4 grams percent to 2.4 grams percent and was supported. At forty-eight hours (about two days), the level was 2.2 grams percent. His general status improved.

The effect of TNS on the underlying pathology other than the hypotension has yet to be appreciated. Further TNS infusions were not a component of his ongoing medical treatment plan.

His improvement was moderate, the ileus resolved, and feedings were adequate. He was returned to his prehospital status. He was discharged on his home ventilator support, parenteral insulin with glucose testing, and a modified oral diet.

Discussion: TNS, a new albumin product formed via the compounding of a mixture of human serum albumin and hydrolyzed amino acids in normal saline, supplied a new tool in management of hypovolemia and circulatory compromise.

The volume benefit was very nonspecific, and the improvement was better perfusion. His responsiveness returned and he just looked better.

His very low serum albumin increased and were maintained. This was a different response with TNS when this pattern was compared to albumin treatment alone. Correction of hypoalbuminemia was not yet a treatment goal of treatment with TNS therapy.

Conclusion: TNS a new albumin product formed via the compounding of a mixture of human serum albumin and hydrolyzed amino acids in normal saline provided a new tool in management of medical pathophysiology of hypovolemia and incidentally increased the serum albumin.

Miracle Case Number Six

This patient was a nineteen-year-old who, one week after a normal pregnancy and delivery, developed a severe autoimmune vasculitis following the birth of her first child.

She initially presented with a high fever, shock, and prominent inflammatory activity signs. She was immediately transferred from the emergency department to a regional tertiary care center.

This research hospital provided very aggressive diagnostic and therapeutic measures. The working diagnosis was juvenile dermatomyositis.

The acute high dose steroid treatment and antibody infusions did not control her disease. Experimental medications (not listed) did not staunch the progressively downhill course of what was then diagnosed as refractory juvenile dermatomyositis.

This patient had a rapidly deteriorating course with severe weakness.

She was unable to manage her baby's visit. Her weakness was so extreme she was unable to even sit in bed.

A frank discussion with the patient and her parents ensued about the futility of further treatment was conducted by the tertiary hospital medical staff.

The consensus of the conference was that she had exhausted all the known available treatment modalities. No other treatment options were available. Everyone present accepted that the therapy was futile she was going to die.

Her medical management problems were made even more difficult by the long distance from her home. A program of supportive (terminal) care at a local hospital PICU was finally arranged.

Arrangements were completed and she was admitted to the local PICU. The local hospital made an exception to allow for terminal supportive care within the PICU. Medical care was to be limited to supportive measures because maximal hospital benefit had been achieved.

She was transported for continuation of only supportive terminal care, which would be provided at this site much closer to her baby and family.

The goal of the accepting medical team in the PICU was to make her global situation better if possible. Those essential medical support items all would be continued.

Her program consisted of total parenteral nutrition (TPN), IV steroids, and every third-day albumin infusion for treatment of severe hypoalbuminemia.

TNS was available at this hospital. TNS was deemed a better alternative treatment agent for correction of hypoalbuminemia. The infusions of TNS 600 ml (about 20.29 oz) increased her albumin levels into the low normal range and controlled her edema.

Surprisingly, the program of every third-day albumin changed when TNS was used. TNS kept the serum albumin levels over 2.0 gram percent. TNS was the clinically appropriate medical therapy in this hospital.

TNS infusions were extended to every three-week interval and given only when her albumin was low. As her albumin levels increased so did her strength, along with increased activity and interest in life.

Amazingly, she gained strength and gradually was able to sit in bed. She could now help with her own oral feedings. The TPN became unnecessary. She was well enough to eat and meet her needs.

Her treatments for juvenile dermatomyositis were continued unchanged.

Most importantly, she had enough strength to hold her baby for the first time. Her recovery course was amazing, and even more amazing considering her severe autoimmune disease was poorly controlled.

She developed enough strength to sit up in a wheelchair for long durations and was able to hold and feed her infant.

This progress continued and a home therapy program with care provided by her mother and sisters was developed.

This "terminal care stay" lasted for about three months until she was able to leave this hospital.

This maintenance of the normal serum albumin levels altered her disease course somehow.

Her course was steady improvement in her ability to feed orally and she gradually begin physical therapy. The clinical goals were to get her into a wheelchair and to be able to hold her baby. Prior to this change, she had not been strong enough to do anything with her baby. Each infusion period seemed to benefit her.

She was discharged to home care with her medical support program to care for her and also to provide care for her infant. This was a successful treatment plan. Medications for continued treatment of her juvenile dermatomyositis were continued. Follow-up appointments were scheduled. Discharge was such a happy day for everyone, especially our staff who had worked so closely with her.

Follow-up did not occur! She was the classic "lost to follow up" patient. Despite social services and home health nursing, contact was totally lost. The patient never returned. She and her family could not be found using everything at our disposal.

Hospital gossip eventually provided the only information. After eight weeks (about two months) at home, the manifestations of her autoimmune disease recurred. The patient refused to return to the hospital and died at home. She died at home because she had been told she was certainly going to die of her disease, so she refused to come back to the hospital. Everyone was saddened by that piece of social gossip. Confirmation of any of these details was never obtained.

Her life in our hospital was very important. TNS corrected her hypoalbuminemia when albumin alone had never done so. That is a minor breakthrough in medical history.

She was never chosen to get TNS. She needed proteins to keep her comfortable. Her remarkable improvement was just a miracle. The concern she would die and the TNS would be blamed was never a consideration. If she had died, the review would have caused problems, taken time, and probably doomed TNS. Her improvement was a needed miracle that saved TNS.

The development plan for TNS was carefully developed to avoid any violations of hospital rules, regulations, and by-laws. All ethics guidance and regulations were reviewed, assessed, and conscientiously accepted, and full compliance was assured. Only after this tedious work to ensure complete compliance on all accounts was the use of TNS planned. No shortcuts or excuses could be permitted.

The severe chronic hypoalbuminemia has never been a treatable disease. Her very good response seems to be the most dramatic recorded. Her disease-specific medical treatments were continued for juvenile dermatomyositis. She seemed to have controlled her autoimmune disease, but that could not be confirmed.

This case showed control of hypoalbuminemia could be done. How this may change recovery from so many different conditions will need to be studied. How much, if any, of her recovery was due to

TNS. She and her amazing responses rewarded our efforts and keeps us committed to pursuing the search for the cure.

Our humanistic care provided her with the strength to mother her child and to interact with her family. The time TNS allowed her to be a mother to her infant was unbelievably valuable.

Upon review of her medical care, the use of the TNS was the single change of the medical treatments that differed from the tertiary care center. The serum albumin levels were pushed to normal, and when normal levels occurred, her edema was modified and her tissue perfusion improved. She began to eat and be more active. No assessment of her primary disease was permitted, but subjectively she was much improved.

How did this happen? What was the mechanism that helped the severely chronically ill patient? This case is remarkable, as all prior interventions had helped very little. TPN was maintained within the circulation and provided circulatory support. Whether a role for suppression of her inflammatory response was present could not be determined.

Something more than an adjustment in the serum albumin had happened.

TNS had very different benefits, correcting and maintaining normal albumin levels within the circulation. (Standard albumin had not been maintained within the circulation). **Subjectively, her refractory juvenile dermatomyositis seemed to be less severe, but the clinically applied limits (rules for hospital acceptance) precluded repeated laboratory studies.**

What role did TNS play in this complex disease state? The TNS role seems to have been a reason for the dramatic reversal from progress to death to a functional mother. Did it play a role? This reversal of this rare autoimmune disease has not been seen before.

Miracle Case Number Seven

A fourteen-year-old boy from Honduras was brought to the hospital emergency department by Border Patrol officers. For the past unknown number of days (five at least) he had experienced severe abdominal pain and had been unable to keep food down. No other history was available, as he was an unaccompanied illegal alien.

On emergency department admission, he was extremely dehydrated and very anorexic, but he was still alert and responsive. Pulse was 130. Blood pressure was 90/45. Peripheral perfusion was poor. Eyes were sunken, mucus membranes were dry, and the skin showed tenting. The ears, nose, and throat were dry but normal. The chest exam was clear. No cardiac murmurs were present. The abdomen was hard and very tender with reflex guarding. The rest of the exam was generally normal. His admission diagnosis was ruptured appendix with generalized peritonitis, septic shock, and severe dehydration.

Lactated Hartmann's solution (5000 milliliters (about 1.32 gal)) was given for initial fluid resuscitation. Broad-spectrum antibiotics (piperacillin and cefuroxime) were started.

The patient was stabilized before being brought to the operating room.

Upon opening the abdomen, a ruptured appendix with peritonitis and multiple abscesses were found. The appendix was removed, and the peritoneal space was copiously irrigated. Primary wound closure was carried out.

The postoperative course was difficult. His fever persisted for the next nine days. Ileus persisted and five repeat abdominal explorations were needed to drain multiple abscesses.

Total parenteral nutrition was required even after the ninth day. Even small amounts of clear liquids could not be tolerated. The patient had a generalized toxic course with night sweats and high-spiking fevers. The white blood cell count was elevated. The hemoglobin levels were low and the albumin level was low.

A decision to correct the hypoproteinemia led to a transfusion of 1500 ml (about 50.72 oz (about 1.5 L)) of TNS daily for four days.

The fever resolved, his pulse decreased, perfusion improved, and the ileus (nonworking intestine) resolved rapidly. The vomiting stopped and a regular diet was tolerated. The patient was discharged five days after the initiation of the TNS.

The change in his clinical status was remarkable. It started when TNS was begun. All signs of systemic toxicity resolved far more rapidly than anticipated.

The patient was discharged five days after TNS was given, but this patient was lost to follow-up.

Miracle Case Number Eight

The patient was a fifteen-month-old male who was undergoing chemotherapy for testicular myeloid sarcoma.

He presented with high fever with severe immunosuppressed status.

His hemoglobin was 10.1, 400 white blood cell count, neutrophil count was 0, lymphocyte count was 92 percent, platelet count was 60,000. Sodium 127, Potassium 3.3, Bicarbonate was 16, total protein was 5.6 gram percent, and the serum albumin 3.4 grams percent.

The patient immediately started on broad-spectrum antibiotic treatment and acute volume support with 20 ml. per kg of normal saline for volume resuscitation to improve perfusion.

Over the next week, he developed severe ARDS requiring full ventilator support. Additional fluid volume was given in addition to the current standard of therapy.

The primary manifestations of the inflammatory cascade were refractory, and third Spacing of fluid and severe ARDS were the most difficult to manage. The abnormal hematologic parameters were attributed to chemotherapy. Coagulopathy did not develop. Renal function and liver function were preserved.

At one week of treatment, the patient was quite edematous and required full ventilator support with machine pressure setting of peak pressure of twenty-seven and a mean airway pressure of fifteen. All attempts to wean his ventilator support failed. his chest X-ray showed a pattern of ARDS or pulmonary edema.

Fluid overload was refractory to diuretic treatment. Weight had increased from 15.83 kg on admission to 17.1 kg on the day prior to treatment with TNS.

Weight on the morning of day one of treatment was 18.8 kg. Ventilator settings were unchanged. Laboratory studies were normal, as were electrolytes and renal function and liver function, serum albumin was 2.4 gm percent.

The treatment program continued all current therapies without modification, with the addition of TNS at 15ml/kg administered over two hours, and repeated every twelve hours. Serum albumin was 3.3 grams percent on the second day of TNS treatments.

Weight at onset was 18.8 kg; day one- 16 kg and at day two-15 kg. His weight remained at the admission level until discharge.

Respiratory status improved very rapidly, and the patient was weaned progressively and extubated to nasal cannula on the third day; a dramatic change from his prior status.

The remainder of the hospital course was very benign, and the chemotherapy treatment protocols were resumed.

This is a very different course of recovery and a remarkably different rate of recovery than anyone had seen before. Most remarkable was the clearing of the infiltrates and resumption of near-normal breathing in a very short period. The fluid overload status had been refractory for one week, but with the TNS it resolved in two days. The post-ventilator respiratory tract problems were minimal.

This is an example of the very significant changes in the disease process that occur after the introduction of TNS into the treatment program.

TNS appears to benefit the vascular integrity, which can only be done when the glycocalyx layer of the endothelium is functional.

No other product has ever done these remarkable physiologic changes.

Fortunately, the changes in the disease course in each and every patient were remarkable. The rapid recovery from fluid overload. The prevention and the resolutions of the fever did not match anticipated responses. Something very different was uncovered and shown in these few illustrative cases.

More studies and more reports must be generated. But up to this time **no other treatment mode has ever changed the clinical course so dramatically.**

Once the beneficial effects were noted, the staff looked for all others who could benefit.

A group of patients with low serum albumin levels was selected. TNS was administered, and less dramatic responses were documented, but a new phenomenon became apparent: TNS could correct low albumin levels.

A prospective treatment program was established to identify and treat all patients in this PICU who had abnormally low serum albumin levels. This was a medical treatment program, not a study group.

When the albumin was abnormal (at less than 2.5 gram percent) these patients were treated with 15 ml/kg (about 0.51 oz) for three doses every eight or twelve hours.

Patients were consecutively entered into the treatment group. No patient was omitted for any reason. The medical diagnosis was random and varied in severity.

Twenty-five consecutively identified patients with albumin levels less than 2.5 gm percent were treated.

All twenty-five patients had improvement in tested laboratory values, and the serum albumin levels increased into the normal range in all. In all the treated patients, the serum albumin levels continued to increase over the next three to five days.

Hypoalbuminemia corrected in all twenty-five patients. TN response occurred across all pediatric ages and varied diagnoses.

Importantly, no adverse incidents or problems occurred.

The patients seemed to recover more quickly, and all were discharged home within four days despite widely varied diagnoses. The patients "seemed" to be much improved.

No comparable series is available for comparison.

In 1970 hypoalbuminemia was reported to correlate with increased mortality and death. Hypoalbuminemia has continuously been associated with significantly increased mortality and morbidity for all patients regardless of diagnosis and age.

The problem with hypoalbuminemia has persisted without change until now.

The historical studies of albumin infusions exhibited a pattern of a failure to correct low albumin levels and after infusion of albumin all promptly returned to their low pretreatment albumin levels. The many similar studies of hypoalbuminemia all confirm the infusion treatment failure.

These 25 TNStreated cases demonstrate very different pathophysiologic responses. These results are compared to standard human serum albumin treatments in many other studies published in the literature.

Clinical conclusions from the TNS infusion study are:

- Volume overload resolved promptly and safely.
- Fluid overload did not occur with TNS treatments at 15 ml/kg.
- Inflammatory responses were suppressed in all patients.
- Hypoalbuminemia was corrected and maintained on all patients with use of TNS.

The recognition of the subtleties in the disease presentation and course provided the original basis for the observations.

This whole line of pathophysiologic change resulted from the observations of an experienced critical care physician. The clinical conditions changed after TNS was administered both in the sick and hypoalbuminemic patients.

These are clinical observations of successful healing outcomes of the sepsis syndrome with TNS.

The Conclusion: (derived from these clinical observations) The Norberg Solution—TNS is a compounded albumin and amino acid product that interferes and blocks the inflammatory cascade progress to directly benefit the patient.

TNS is the first of a new class of products that directly blocks the inflammatory cascade disease progression within the patient.

TNS starts a new paradigm in medicine: Treating the patient itself!

This new paradigm builds on established treatments and uses the concept of EGLX repair using TNS as a substrate.

These are direct clinical observations of modified differences in the disease pathophysiology after TNS treatment. These cases establish the basis for treating sepsis with TNS infusions.

This starts a new paradigm in medicine; all older treatments work to keep disease from invading the patient. These old treatment tools are focused on treating the infecting problem before sepsis and septic shock start; after sepsis nothing could be done.

It is correct to treat the causes traditionally. But when the sepsis becomes established in the patient, treat the patient with TNS to stop the sepsis.

TNS treatments act directly to help the patient stop this deadly process and heal themselves.. These treatments work to stop sepsis within the patient.

This pattern of response is totally new and different from our experience and training. TNS—an albumin and amino acid compound provides substrate into the patient to facilitate the patient's recovery.

All patients treated with TNS improved! All patients survived and recovered.

There were no adverse effects.

TNS begins a new paradigm in medical treatment today! TNS is medical albumin product with benefits never before observed.

TNS directly benefits the patient! Nothing else has ever directly helped patients by interfering with sepsis.

To all physicians: This is a complete radical paradigm shift.

You can do TNS treatments.

You can directly observe this miracle in your own patients.

You will save lives!

You will witness this miraculous response, by yourself and in your saved patients.!

TNS is a safe new and beneficial treatment here today and bringing in a new paradigm.

Tomorrow has been changed forever!!

CHAPTER TEN

A Miracle in Modern Medicine

TNS is **The Norberg Solution,** a modified albumin amino acid mixture in normal saline with no additional components. Nomenclature is in the classic manner; Ringer's solution, Hartmann's solution, and now Norberg's solution.

TNS production is allowed by the Law Summary: ***S.959 — 113th Congress (2013-2014).*** This comprehensive legislative act clearly spells out all the details required for compounded products:

> USA production standards used in the preparation are found in public published references. USP Pharmacopeial; chapter 797 and ISO f Regulations for Facilities Class 5,7 & 8. These are used within the USA. These can be referenced and correlated with each individual country's regulations. These are basic hygiene requirements for compounded products.

Recently published FDA guidelines are available, ***Mixing Diluting, or Repackaging Biological Products Outside the Scope of an Approved Biologics License Application Guidance for Industry*** US Department of Health and Human Services, Food and Drug Administration, Center for Drug Evaluation and Research (CDER), Center for Biologics Evaluation and Research (CBER), January 1, 2018. Compounding and Related Documents.

Before discussing the implications of TNS, pharmaceutical information about TNS is provided.

TNS has no chemical interaction as albumin has no chemical activity, hydrolyzed amino acid solutions have no intrinsic chemical activity, and these products in combination are chemically inactive.

The albumin is a long continuous chain of amino acids that is folded into a commonly illustrated pattern that is the known and accepted physiologic configuration.

Amino acids are individual molecules of all amino acids. This mixture is stable.

A specific protein analysis by a school of pharmacy laboratory showed no agglutination, polymerization, no precipitation, and the polydispersity essentially unchanged from the natural albumin alone. Molecular size was increased by 17 percent. Long-term stability testing was not performed.

Human serum albumin is a USA FDA-approved product with a more than seventy-year history of safety in human use. Albumin has no allergic or immunologic problems (human source).

Hydrolyzed amino acids have fifty-plus years of human medical use with no safety issues.

TNS is an inactive metabolically stable protein product originally created to combat the permeability assumed to be leading to the third spacing component of the sepsis syndrome.

The studies presented are the successful result of spontaneous extensive bureaucratic developments resulting in change. The Federal Drug Administration allows the prescription of approved products for compounding when prescribed by the treating physician and formulated by the pharmacist in a safe and secure manner. This is the key regulatory change.

Human serum albumin and hydrolyzed amino acids are basic hospital pharmacy and blood bank products readily available in all major hospitals. Albumin and amino acid solutions are standard pharmacy inventory.

The compounding process is simple. Most hospitals are using the sterile airflow hood apparatus generally present in all major hospitals. This is a simple mixture that does not require any additional steps. Sterility must always be maintained. The albumin mixture does not require refrigeration. The studies needed to determine the safe shelf life of the product have not been performed. Current recommendations that TNS be used within twenty-four to forty-eight hours of production.

This compounded product can be mixed by all medical facilities throughout the entire world. The basic formulary: human serum albumin to a 5 percent concentration and hydroxylated amino acids to a 2 percent concentration in normal saline with no other mineral or other compounds added. State-of-the-art procedures are assumed to be followed to ensure sterility.

Pricing and availability are not problems, as these products are already known. The equipment and the skilled personnel are universally present. These ubiquitous factors make TNS available to all hospitals for the treatment of the sepsis syndrome.

This is a breakthrough miracle available to our entire world and begins a new paradigm in medicine!

How can TNS work?

The patient with sepsis receives all standard therapies for sepsis. Following initiation of these treatments, TNS dosing can be started, and dosage is based on the clinician's decision. For pediatric patients ,15-20 ml per kg seems a good starting point. If perfusion deficits are noted, repeated dosing should be performed. Adult dosing generally follows the same pattern, but since each unit of albumin, is within the needed volume the whole unit should be mixed and administered. Repeat the TNS dose as the patient's status indicates need.

The perfusion should increase, and blood pressure should gradually normalize. The inflammatory responses gradually diminish. Most apparent was the fever resolution. In no patient in this series did coagulopathy manifest. No patient developed ARDS, but one patient had an improved course of his ARDS with TNS. So, no ARDS-related conclusions should be made.

The worst-case scenario is a poor response to the volume loading and continued perfusion failure. As with crystalloid, additional volume is given (TNS has no adverse reactions) so may be continued. Vasopressor therapy can be added.

Severe destruction of the entire EGLX may have occurred. Recovery may not be possible when the EGLX function has been destroyed or paralyzed. TNS cannot resuscitate a dead EGLX. More research on this aspect of sepsis and treatment is needed.

Theoretical answer to "Why this product works"

The question is: Should any mechanism be proposed with so little data? The answer is obviously NO, but that never stops anyone. Speculation time! There is no scientific basis at all for the mechanism of action at present.

The albumin molecule as described is a tight-bound integrated folded long string of 585 amino acid molecules bound together with covalent binding at some sites and at other sites bound by ligand binding.

My first primitive explanation is: TNS is a newly separated processed blood product. Albumin studies seem to indicate that covalent bonding molecules (magnesium and calcium) contribute to the described albumin molecule configuration. When albumin is confronted by the varied amino acids, these amino acids are incorporated into the tangled mass of the albumin in a passive manner, but probably not in any specific pattern. This increases the size by 17 percent.

This albumin molecule could be more available for metabolic and structural repair.

No data supports any pattern as an explanation for the change in size of this albumin molecule. The current new molecular visualization studies will certainly help find these answers quickly. Now is the time to start to look.

More speculation: These combinations could result in a new and different molecule with a cotton candy-like form. This soft molecule could be captured by the break in the surface of the glycocalyx and then effectively covers the damaged site, or it can be pulled into the damaged by electromagnetic forces known to be present at that site. TNS becomes an essential substrate used to repair the damaged EGLX layer.

You can make up your own answer and it probably will be better answer. This whole field is open to everyone to make their discoveries.

The whole area of sepsis intervention is now wide open for development. There's never been anything like this! Anticipate a virtual Gold Rush scenario!

This mechanism is now only a point of speculation that will be addressed and answered in the years to come.

This area is rife for discovery. This revelation should make the California Gold Rush of 1849 seem slow!

TNS is different! A new paradigm in medicine has arrived.

There is nothing ever known to have this unique effect on human disease.

TNS is for all.

CHAPTER ELEVEN

TNS is Here! Bring it to the Fight to End Sepsis!

TNS is the ultimate manifestation of the medical miracle of the twenty-first century.

YOU STILL HAVE TO MAKE THE MIRACLE HAPPEN!

This chapter is the review and culmination of all the information presented. This is the truth in research statement.

All the background for the questions that arise has been presented as directly and honestly as possible. In some discussions lack of data is the problem, and in other situations a limited understanding may affect the degree of completeness. Decision criteria was "reasonable medical certainty." This essentially is patient treatment decision-making.

All data and statements are presented in an honest and ethical manner. No deviations from best practices and current medical ethics have occurred in the development of TNS.

This book presents the best effort of the author to conquer the problem of sepsis that has plagued medicine forever. Sepsis may eventually kill us unless we make the changes needed.

The source of this conclusion is the result of clinical care of individual patients; not all patients who received TNS were included.

Each person, even those who must not be recognized, did contribute to the development of TNS. This clinical information was combined into the known scientific milieu to formulate TNS.

Only a small number of patient care cases have been presented. All clinical information was obtained from post-treatment discharge reports in the medical records. In some cases, the medical record was not available and patient outcomes remained unknown. This is due to very strict adherence to the restrictions regarding privacy maintenance in the performance of post-discharge medical record review.

No known ethical guidelines were ever violated or "stretched." For example, special instructions could not be given to the bedside nurse to alter or even better comply with patient weight routines or ask for better documentation.

All patients received TNS only as an indicated medical therapy. The observations are limited by incomplete medical charting. Only the standard laboratory studies for their disease were able to be performed, no special interventions or special follow-up studies were permitted at any point for any patient.

What was there is all there is here.

Still, some consistent unique observations could be made:

1. Fluid mobilization occurred when diuretics failed.

2. Third spacing seemed to be prevented.

3. Serum albumin levels uniformly improved and persisted.

4. Febrile reactions and inflammatory responses seemed to be minimalized or absent.

5. Sepsis and septic shock responded to moderate volumes of TNS.

6. TNS did not appear to be involved in third spacing.

7. Fluid volumes needed for resuscitation appeared to be less than crystalloid fluid volumes.

8. No changes in renal function were recorded as measured by BUN and creatine.

9. This grouping did not include patients likely to die.

10. No complications or worsening occurred in any patient treated.

This patient grouping did not include patients likely to die. This subset of patients was felt likely to interfere and possibly compromise TNS use and development. The actuality was that some patients had a high degree of severity of their illness and were transferred to a tertiary center to receive specific technical interventions. Their illness course was not known, and no comparison of the disease course and their outcomes could be made.

The reality was that no patient was ever refused TNS.

No adverse incidents ever happened.

Ignaz Semmelweis commented that the illnesses were different even when there was no obvious reason for any difference to be present.

The pattern of EGLX injury and the patterns of inflammatory reactions leading to fever, increased white blood cell counts, lower platelet counts, coagulopathy or bleeding, systemic reaction, organ dysfunction, and central nervous system failure; the responses were all changed after treatment with TNS.

The previous discussion of the CHAOS theory to account for the variation in disease presentation as the EGLX undergoes widely variable injury in the area damaged, the depth of the damage and the changing injury accompanying the insult is an important concept.

The glycocalyx can be imagined to be like a blanket of skin and the disease like a rash, pimple, vesicles, or a full-thickness injury, and the area involved in the injury can be of any size and depth; anything goes.

The range of each injury component can vary from very minimal to total EGLX disruption. The injury to the glycocalyx can be a minimal disruption to very deep and severe destructive damage up to and including the death of the endothelial cells. It must be accepted that a state of injury and destruction can be so severe that nothing will alter that course leading directly to the patient's death. Experience over time will clarify these patterns.

The sepsis disease process initially starts when the glycocalyx is damaged and the cytokine storm begins. The gross and microscopic damage may be different, and the resultant cytokine reaction is varied depending upon the individual products released from that site and the intensity of the cascade that results.

This is best explained as **chaos!**

When total endothelial cell dysfunctions due to cell paralysis or cell death, the cell interfaces allow extracellular fluid to be lost freely into the subcutaneous tissues unrestricted, which may cause an injury that cannot be healed. This injury leads to the death of the patient.

This explanation for the wide range of severity of the illness manifested during sepsis is reasonable. But the theory is not yet proven.

TNS is such a different product than any previously used in medicine. No compounds, whether herbal, vegetarian, fungal, jungle plants, or even Chinese herbal products have demonstrated these or similar physiologic functional changes in the human.

The administration of TNS allowed the changes in the pathophysiology to be observed, The interpretations of these changes were used to expand our knowledge about the inflammatory cascade and sepsis.

TNS is truly the first product ever to be able to beneficially access (support) the glycocalyx layer and change the sepsis syndrome. This brings new information to us and changes our perspective on sepsis.

The infusion of TNS had no additional pathologic conditions developed or progressed after treatment. This indicates that the developing and expanding components of sepsis were stopped or modified by TNS administration. Whatever the difference, TNS is metabolically and physiologically accessible to block the enzyme cascade that occurs within the glycocalyx layer.

TNS brings a physiologic action that seemingly allows the EGLX actions to be modified. The inflammatory reaction seems to have had its severity decreased and some of the disease processes stopped. These are clinical observations and further experience will better define these actions. But these are good starting places.

The existing correlation between low serum proteins and poor clinical outcomes and increased mortality has been general medical knowledge since 1970. This hypoalbuminemia has been refractory to all interventions (primarily albumin transfusions). Transfusion with albumin does not correct the problem. This is present at all ages and all diseases.

Transfusion with TNS does correct the low proteins in a very small pediatric patient group. Large studies over time will be needed to determine whether correction of the low protein levels will change the mortality and morbidity. Low protein levels and a thinner glycocalyx layer have been recorded as being associated with illness and aging. But there is no convincing data to support this relationship. TNS infusion causes a physiologic increase in albumin levels that natural albumin does not cause. In the cases following TNS transfusion, every patient had an increased albumin level that persisted.

The intravascular persistence of TNS in the circulatory system is longer than albumin, but the half-life of TNS could not be estimated. Caregivers reported soft tissues were firmer and well-perfused when compared to the intercurrent illness and were "of better quality."

Albumin correction does not correct low albumin levels in ill patients even with full metabolic support. The fluid dynamics are simply different, circulatory stability and perfusion was far better following TNS.

The specific anti-inflammatory interaction of TNS, presumably with leukotrienes, is only an observed clinical response. But in all cases systemic toxicity decreased.

The disease state was definitely modified by TNS, and all patients appeared to have a milder form of illness with a shorter length of illness.

The length of time for glycocalyx recovery cannot even be estimated from this very limited data if glycocalyx recovery is what is the observed physiologic response.

At this point, conclusions must be made. A wholly new concept of disease is revealed here. The definition of sepsis has been amplified, a mechanism of the inflammatory cascade been modified, and a novel product (TNS) is directly involved in providing constituents (substrates) to the healing process within the glycocalyx.

TNS is the first-ever product that directly provides a means of controlling or correcting the sepsis process within the human body.

All prior medical programs have been directed to the elimination of the inciting factor, killing bacteria-stopping viral reproduction.

All the interventions of today occur on the exterior of the human disease stage once the disease entered the human host. Only the host's own defenses affect the recovery.

TNS TREATS THE PATIENT DIRECTLY!

NOTHING ELSE HAS EVER DONE ANYTHING TO SUPPORT THE DYING PATIENT'S DISEASE STATE!

Future studies will clarify the exact mechanics of TNS action. Whether it is interference or repair of the glycocalyx layer, a definite alteration of the destructive sepsis cascade happens and is more readily incorporated into the repair or restoration. This will certainly be a focus of future research.

A critical look into the molecular action is likely to lead to the development of more and different products to "help" the glycocalyx layer in its functional recovery. TNS opens the door to a whole new paradigm of disease control products.

TNS is the first product in all of time that directly helps the patient dying of sepsis!

All other medical therapies focus on killing the pathogen and leaving the patient alone to survive or die.

Our medical future will be different after TNS introduction. TNS opens the door to the vast new area of glycocalyx research and new discoveries.

When your endothelial glycocalyx organ is damaged your illness begins; and when the EGLX returns to normal, your illness ends!

How could life become more exciting?

CHAPTER TWELVE

Enter a New Paradigm in the Treatment of Sepsis!

THE INFLAMMATORY CASCADE STARTS WHEN THE EGLX IS DAMAGED.

THE DISEASE STATE ENDS WHEN THE EGLX RETURNS TO NORMAL.

This is the new inflammatory theory needed to understand sepsis.

Where to from here?

The future is so important to us.

There is an old story about a psychic woman who sells a crystal ball to a customer, and at the end of the transaction says, "Use it in good health, doctor."

When the woman is asked how in the world could she know the customer was a doctor, she replies, "Doctors are the only people so focused on the future."

The future will come whether we like it or not. We can either do something to make that future and everyone's lives better, or we can do nothing and allow future generations to continue to suffer needlessly.

The Norberg Solution (TNS) is the first medical product ever developed that changes the pathophysiology responses in sepsis. TNS is a simple combination mixture of human serum albumin and hydrolyzed amino acid solution in normal saline solution. It is so unique a product, despite its simplicity, that it was granted a patent by the United States Patent Office. This combination product production is permitted under the combination rules of the Federal Drug Administration (FDA) in the USA.

Human serum albumin is FDA-approved without restriction for human use. No warnings or restrictions are provided to users. It has been safely used since 1941. Hydrolyzed amino acid solution has been safely used in total parenteral nutrition support since 1955. No warnings or limitations are placed upon either product.

The albumin and amino acids are uniformly available in all major hospital pharmacies at a reasonable cost. The process of mixing is simple following the sterility rules established for the preparation of the TPN products.

TNS provides a metabolically available albumin molecule, presumably to the damaged EGLX layer. Mechanisms of this action are only theoretically provided. So much more must be done, but exciting changes will undoubtedly happen as its use continues.

These simple reasonable facts make TNS available to almost every treating physician in the entire world. Nothing like this has ever occurred before, and physicians have the unique opportunity to be a part of this innovative new solution to the plague of sepsis that has taken the lives of far too many patients who could have survived and thrived if TNS had been available to them.

The future of lifesaving sepsis treatment is about to begin. Where will you be when it happens?

Two actual articles from current medical publications describe the status of sepsis treatment today (November 2022). The *Journal of the American Medical Association (JAMA)* (September 2022) issue includes a current sepsis case report, as does *The Critical Care Medical Journal* (December 2022 issue), which includes a case report of current sepsis management.

Each of these medical journal presentations showcases the full impact of sepsis on the patient, who dies; the family, who suffers; the medical care providers, who are devastated by the loss; and the critical care specialist, who knows the care given to the patient was the best available but in the end proved to be inadequate.

Please compare these outcomes of best care today to the new concept of treatment with TNS. The few similar cases presented in this book have different outcomes and bring a new promise of hope to all caregivers.

These are the reasons for working in the long search to "Find a Cure for Sepsis."

A medical case is presented as an "avatar" (a fact-based story) to show the status of medicine treatments today. This story brings an understanding of the author's medical career providing critical care, always struggling against SEPSIS. Cases like these determined the need and provided the continuing incentive to do the work that was involved in

In the article "Finding the Cure for Sepsis," The author uses their experience as a medical professional providing critical care to examine the struggle against sepsis using an avatar (fact-based story) of a typical patient struggling with sepsis. Cases like the one in this article perfectly demonstrate the desperate need and continuing incentive to find a way to cure this insidious condition.

The article begins by entering the room to evaluate a six-month-old male infant very ill with a fever. The exam shows that the baby is sufferi9ng from meningitis with a full anterior fontanelle, with the high-pitched cry and an unmistakable Brudzinski sign shown when his neck is flexed. A lumbar puncture is the key test, and he gives only a feeble cry for a moment. The fluid is cloudy, confirming that this is the correct diagnosis.

The treatment program is well known and how such cases are handled in hospitals around the world every day. First, antibiotics and steroids are immediately employed, followed by intubation under sedation. During the procedures described in this article, petechiae are noted, and bleeding and bruises are showing all over. This is purpura fulminans. Death is coming, and while the whole team caring for this infant can do many things, there will be no stopping this disease. Everyone sees it coming. The family also sees the changes and are in a state of disbelief and weeping as they watch their baby son, whose life had been so full of promise and a horizon of tomorrows, slowly die despite the medical team's best efforts.

The team develops a unique bond, providing support for each other while focused on this baby and his family. The tiny body begins to seize, as is so common with this disease. The team works to control the seizure, but it is bad.

The CT scanner is such a huge machine, and this tiny child looks even more so when he is placed into it to get the scan. This study must be done immediately to be certain nothing treatable is overlooked.

On the return to his room, he barely resembles the infant who was admitted into the hospital the previous night. He is incredibly ill and seems to lack the life force.

Death is clearly coming for this baby soon, and the small team of doctors and nurses tries to keep the family present and give the loving care they so desperately need. The treatment could not have been better, and everyone is strongly supported for the role they each played.

The CT and ultrasound confirm the team's worst fears; the baby has suffered brain death and there is nothing more they can do.

The absolute confirmation of the death is presented to the parents, and the baby is removed from all medical support items and lovingly wrapped in a blanket for his final journey to the morgue.

The mother holds her precious son for the last time; tears running silently down her face. His father is present but in a different fatherly way, he walks around the room and thanks the staff and suffers his sadness stoically. The medical team supports this family well; they are good at doing that. What we as medical professionals are not good at is preventing death!

The post-death review confirms what the team already knew. From this situation and many others in many other places, the determination is developed to find something that will stop this disease.

There truly was nothing available to help this poor child. Tomorrow will be the same! Unless . . .

My answer to this urgent need for a new therapy is TNS.

I have developed TNS, a product that can be given to a patient to help fight the disease called sepsis. TNS opens a door to focus on a search for new therapies that will directly help the patient.

TNS appears to stop sepsis; but much more work is still to be done.

Penicillin kills the bacteria and leaves the patient alone, unharmed by the drug. There has never been anything that improved the patient's ability to tolerate sepsis and repair the body from the ravages of sepsis. TNS seems to be a paradigm shift that will change all of medicine.

I believe our future will be different. With TNS, my dream and goal is that each patient who suffers from sepsis receives a TNS-like treatment and lives to see a recovery to good health every time.

TNS is the first breakthrough into the new world of sepsis treatment. Hopefully, the difficulties of adopting other major discoveries will not become a part of the TNS story of curing sepsis.

TNS is the miracle answer to the prayers of every doctor who has ever stood helplessly by as their patient died of a disease that could not be stopped or even understood.

This is the new paradigm.

The breakthrough sepsis cure has arrived in our lifetimes.

TNS is the first.

This just the beginning.

Come along, do and see the miracles!

Life will be so much better for us all!

Bibliography

This bibliography is an abbreviated list derived from the large number of articles, books, and conferences available. Many were used in the development of this new concept and medical product in treatment of patients with sepsis.

1. Starling, Ernest H. "On the Absorption of Fluids from the Connective Tissue Spaces." *The Journal of Physiology* 19, no. 4 (1896): 312–26. https://doi.org/10.1113/jphysiol.1896.sp000596.

2. Kenny, Jon-Emile S. "The Revised Starling Principle: Implications for Rational Fluid Therapy." PulmCCM. PulmCCM, July 7, 2016. https://www.pulmccm.org/p/revised-starling-principle-implications-rational-fluid-therapy.

3. Schött, Ulf, Cristina Solomon, Dietmar Fries, and Peter Bentzer. "The Endothelial Glycocalyx and Its Disruption, Protection and Regeneration: A Narrative Review." *Scandinavian Journal of Trauma, Resuscitation and Emergency Medicine* 24, no. 1 (2016). https://doi.org/10.1186/s13049-016-0239-y.

4. Moore, Benjamin. "In Memory of Sidney Ringer [1835-1910]." *Biochemical Journal* 5, no. 6-7 (1911). https://doi.org/10.1042/bj005000i.

5. O'Shaughnessy, W.B. "Experiments on the Blood in Cholera." *The Lancet* 17, no. 435 (1831): 490. https://doi.org/10.1016/s0140-6736(02)94389-8.

6. Lewins, Robert, and Rob. Lewins. "Injection of Saline Solutions in Extraordinary Quantities into the Veins in Cases of Malignant Cholera." *The Lancet* 18, no. 456 (1832): 243–44. https://doi.org/10.1016/s0140-6736(02)82831-8.

7. "Tweede Brief Van Den Aertsbisschop Van Sebaste Aan De Katholyke Ingesetenen Van Het Vereenigde Nederland." *Dutch Pamphlets Online*, n.d. https://doi.org/10.1163/2214-8264_dutchpamphlets-kb1-kb18145.

8. Hartmann, Alexis F., and Milton J.E. Senn. "Studies in the Metabolism of Sodium R-Lactate. I. Response of Normal Human Subjects to the Intravenous Injection of Sodium R-Lactate." *Journal of Clinical Investigation* 11, no. 2 (1932): 327–35. https://doi.org/10.1172/jci100414.

9.   "The History of the Army Medical Department." *Journal of the Royal Army Medical Corps* 120, no. 3 (1974): 136–37. https://doi.org/10.1136/jramc-120-03-01.

10. McClelland, DB. "Safety of Human Albumin as a Constituent of Biologic Therapeutic Products." *Transfusion* 38, no. 7 (1998): 690–99. https://doi.org/10.1046/j.1537-2995.1998.38798346639.x.

11. Hartog, Christiane S., Dorit Reuter, Wolfgang Loesche, Michael Hofmann, and Konrad Reinhart. "Influence of Hydroxyethyl Starch (HES) 130/0.4 on Hemostasis as Measured by Viscoelastic Device Analysis: A Systematic Review." *Intensive Care Medicine* 37, no. 11 (2011): 1725–37. https://doi.org/10.1007/s00134-011-2385-z.

12. SL;, Roberts JS;, Bratton. "Colloid Volume Expanders. Problems, Pitfalls and Possibilities." Drugs. U.S. National Library of Medicine. Accessed March 21, 2023. https://pubmed.ncbi.nlm.nih.gov/9585860/.

13. Suzuki, Adriana Stama, and Bruna Thomazelli Berbel. "Pediatric Multiple Organ Dysfunction Syndrome Promising Therapies." *Pediatric Critical Care Medicine* 18, no. 7 (2017): 731. https://doi.org/10.1097/pcc.0000000000001202.

14. Baue, Arthur E., Rodney Durham, and Eugen Faist. "Systemic Inflammatory Response Syndrome (SIRS), Multiple Organ Dysfunction Syndrome (MODS), Multiple Organ Failure (MOF)." *shock* 10, no. 2 (1998): 79–89. https://doi.org/10.1097/00024382-199808000-00001.

15. Fleck, A., Felicity Hawker, P.I. Wallace, Gail Raines, J. Trotter, I. Mca. Ledingham, and K.C. Calman. "Increased Vascular Permeability: A Major Cause of Hypoalbuminemia in Disease and Injury." *The Lancet* 325, no. 8432 (1985): 781–84. https://doi.org/10.1016/s0140-6736(85)91447-3.

16. Hahn, Robert G. "Adverse Effects of Infusion Fluids." *Clinical Fluid Therapy in the Perioperative Setting*, 2016, 262–69. https://doi.org/10.1017/cbo9781316401972.036.

17. Reviewers, C. I., and C. I. Reviewers. "Human Albumin Administration in Critically Ill Patients: Systematic Review of Randomized Controlled Trials   Why Albumin May Not Work." *BMJ* 317, no. 7153 (1998): 235–40. https://doi.org/10.1136/bmj.317.7153.235.

18. Leite, Heitor Pons, Alessandra Vaso Rodrigues da Silva, Simone Brasil

de Oliveira Iglesias, and Paulo Cesar Koch Nogueira. "Serum Albumin Is an Independent Predictor of Clinical Outcomes in Critically Ill Children*." *Pediatric Critical Care Medicine* 17, no. 2 (2016). https://doi.org/10.1097/pcc.0000000000000596.

19. "Serum Albumin Level in Critically Ill Pediatric Patients." *Annals of Clinical and Analytical Medicine* 12, no. 12 (2021). https://doi.org/10.4328/acam.20746.

20. Elman, R. "Serum Albumin Regeneration Following Intravenous Amino-Acids (Hydrolyzed Casein) in Hypoproteinemia Produced by Severe Hemorrhage." *Experimental Biology and Medicine* 43, no. 1 (1940): 14–16. https://doi.org/10.3181/00379727-43-11076.

21. "Serum Albumin Regeneration Following Intravenous Amino-Acids ..." Accessed March 22, 2023. https://journals.sagepub.com/doi/abs/10.3181/00379727-43-11076.

22. Fanali, Gabriella, Alessandra di Masi, Viviana Trezza, Maria Marino, Mauro Fasano, and Paolo Ascenzi. "Human Serum Albumin: From Bench to Bedside." *Molecular Aspects of Medicine* 33, no. 3 (2012): 209–90. https://doi.org/10.1016/j.mam.2011.12.002.

23. Caironi, Pietro, and Luciano Gattinoni. "Proposed Benefits of Albumin from the ALBIOS Trial: A Dose of Insane Belief." *Critical Care* 18, no. 5 (2014). https://doi.org/10.1186/s13054-014-0510-4.

24. Doweiko, John P., and Dominic J. Nompleggi. "Use of Albumin as a Volume Expander." *Journal of Parenteral and Enteral Nutrition* 15, no. 4 (1991): 484–87. https://doi.org/10.1177/0148607191015004484.

25. Angus, Derek C., and Randy S. Wax. "Epidemiology of Sepsis: An Update." *Critical Care Medicine* 29 (2001). https://doi.org/10.1097/00003246-200107001-00035.

26. Carcillo, J. A. "Choice of Fluids for Resuscitation in Children with Severe Infection and Shock." *BMJ* 341, no. sep02 1 (2010): c4546–c4546. https://doi.org/10.1136/bmj.c4546.

27. Rhee, Peter, Elena Koustova, and Hasan B. Alam. "Searching for the Optimal Resuscitation Method: Recommendations for the Initial Fluid Resuscitation of Combat Casualties." *Journal of Trauma: Injury, Infection & Critical Care* 54, no. 5 (2003). https://doi.org/10.1097/01.ta.0000064507.80390.10.

28. Norberg, Åke, Olav Rooyackers, Ralf Segersvärd, and Jan Wernerman. "Leakage of Albumin in Major Abdominal Surgery." *Critical Care* 20, no. 1 (2016). https://doi.org/10.1186/s13054-016-1283-8.

29. Chang, Ronald, and John B. Holcomb. "Choice of Fluid Therapy in the Initial Management of Sepsis, Severe Sepsis, and Septic Shock." *Shock* 46, no. 1 (2016): 17–26. https://doi.org/10.1097/shk.0000000000000577.

30. EMERSON, THOMAS E. "Unique Features of Albumin." *Critical Care Medicine* 17, no. 7 (1989): 690–94. https://doi.org/10.1097/00003246-198907000-00020.

31. Zoellner, H., M. Hofler, R. Beckmann, P. Hufnagl, E. Vanyek, E. Bielek, J. Wojta, A. Fabry, S. Lockie, and B.R. Binder. "Serum Albumin Is a Specific Inhibitor of Apoptosis in Human Endothelial Cells." *Journal of Cell Science* 109, no. 10 (1996): 2571–80. https://doi.org/10.1242/jcs.109.10.2571.

32. Myburgh, J. A. "Fluid Resuscitation in Acute Medicine: What Is the Current Situation?" *Journal of Internal Medicine* 277, no. 1 (2014): 58–68. https://doi.org/10.1111/joim.12326.

33. Mullin, Rick. "Cost to Develop New Pharmaceutical Drug Now Exceeds \$2.5B." Scientific American. Scientific American, November 24, 2014. https://www.scientificamerican.com/article/cost-to-develop-new-pharmaceutical-drug-now-exceeds-2-5b/.

34. "The Federal Register." Federal Register: Request Access. Accessed March 21, 2023. https://www.federalregister.gov/documents/2011/06/21/2011-15344/draft-guidances-for-industry-and-food-and-drug-administration-staff-classification-of-products-as.

35. Mali, Shrikant. "Anaphylaxis during the Perioperative Period." *Anesthesia: Essays and Researches* 6, no. 2 (2012): 124. https://doi.org/10.4103/0259-1162.108286.

36. McClelland, DB. "Safety of Human Albumin as a Constituent of Biologic Therapeutic Products." *Transfusion* 38, no. 7 (1998): 690–99. https://doi.org/10.1046/j.1537-2995.1998.38798346639.x.

37. Hawkins, Joy L. "Maternal Morbidity and Mortality: Anesthetic Causes." *Canadian Journal of Anesthesia/Journal canadien d'anesthésie* 49, no. S1 (2002). https://doi.org/10.1007/bf03018130.

38. "Basic Pharmacokinetic Principles Stephen P. Roush, Pharm.D ... - Pedsccm." Accessed March 22, 2023. http://pedsccm.org/FILE-CABI-NET/Practical/Akron_pdfs/10PHARMA.PDF.

39. Arshed, Sabrina, and Michael R. Pinsky. "Applied Physiology of Fluid Resuscitation in Critical Illness." *Critical Care Clinics* 34, no. 2 (2018): 267–77. https://doi.org/10.1016/j.ccc.2017.12.010.

40. Margarson, M. P., and N. Soni. "Serum Albumin: Touchstone or Totem?" *Anaesthesia* 53, no. 8 (1998): 789–803. https://doi.org/10.1046/j.1365-2044.1998.00438.x.

41. McClelland, DB. "Safety of Human Albumin as a Constituent of Biologic Therapeutic Products." *Transfusion* 38, no. 7 (1998): 690–99. https://doi.org/10.1046/j.1537-2995.1998.38798346639.x.

42. Baue, Arthur E., Rodney Durham, and Eugen Faist. "Systemic Inflammatory Response Syndrome (SIRS), Multiple Organ Dysfunction Syndrome (MODS), Multiple Organ Failure (MOF)." *shock* 10, no. 2 (1998): 79–89. https://doi.org/10.1097/00024382-199808000-00001.

43. Kaddourah, Ahmad, Rajit K. Basu, Stuart L. Goldstein, and Scott M. Sutherland. "Oliguria and Acute Kidney Injury in Critically Ill Children." *Pediatric Critical Care Medicine* 20, no. 4 (2019): 332–39. https://doi.org/10.1097/pcc.0000000000001866.

44. Fleck, A., Felicity Hawker, P.I. Wallace, Gail Raines, J. Trotter, I. Mca. Ledingham, and K.C. Calman. "Increased Vascular Permeability: A Major Cause of Hypoalbuminemia in Disease and Injury." *The Lancet* 325, no. 8432 (1985): 781–84. https://doi.org/10.1016/s0140-6736(85)91447-3.

45. Kielstein, Jan T., and Alexander Zarbock. "Is This the Beginning of the End of Cytokine Adsorption?*." *Critical Care Medicine* 50, no. 6 (2022): 1026–29. https://doi.org/10.1097/ccm.0000000000005509.

46. Hahn, Robert G., and Gordon Lyons. "The Half-Life of Infusion Fluids." *European Journal of Anaesthesiology* 33, no. 7 (2016): 475–82. https://doi.org/10.1097/eja.0000000000000436.

47. Leite, Heitor Pons, Alessandra Vaso Rodrigues da Silva, Simone Brasil de Oliveira Iglesias, and Paulo Cesar Koch Nogueira. "Serum Albumin Is an Independent Predictor of Clinical Outcomes in Critically Ill Children*." *Pediatric Critical Care Medicine* 17, no. 2 (2016). https://doi.org/10.1097/pcc.0000000000000596.

48. Mahabee, ME, Deming DD, Abd -Allah SA, et al: Hypoproteinemia; A Treatable Risk Factor: Serum albumin levels in Critically Ill Pediatric Patients; Influence on Outcome. Poster Presentation A VPS Study; Pediatric Critical Care Colloquium 2015

49. Center for Drug Evaluation and Research. "Provisions That Apply to Human Drug Compounding." U.S. Food and Drug Administration. FDA. Accessed March 22, 2023. https://www.fda.gov/drugs/human-drug-compounding/fdc-act-provisions-apply-human-drug-compounding.

50. Center for Drug Evaluation and Research. "Drug Supply Chain Security Act (DSCSA)." U.S. Food and Drug Administration. FDA. Accessed March 22, 2023. https://www.fda.gov/drugs/drug-supply-chain-integrity/drug-supply-chain-security-act-dscsa.

51. Fanali, Gabriella, Alessandra di Masi, Viviana Trezza, Maria Marino, Mauro Fasano, and Paolo Ascenzi. "Human Serum Albumin: From Bench to Bedside." *Molecular Aspects of Medicine* 33, no. 3 (2012): 209–90. https://doi.org/10.1016/j.mam.2011.12.002.

52. Sinclair, Scott E., William A. Altemeier, Gustavo Matute-Bello, and Emil Y. Chi. "Augmented Lung Injury Due to Interaction between Hyperoxia and Mechanical Ventilation*." *Critical Care Medicine* 32, no. 12 (2004): 2496–2501. https://doi.org/10.1097/01.ccm.0000148231.04642.8d.

53. Tandon, Radhika, and Saied Froghi. "Artificial Liver Support Systems." *Journal of Gastroenterology and Hepatology* 36, no. 5 (2020): 1164–79. https://doi.org/10.1111/jgh.15255.

54. Bartlett, Robert H. "The Origins of Continuous Renal Replacement Therapy." *ASAIO Journal* 64, no. 3 (2018): 427–30. https://doi.org/10.1097/mat.0000000000000573.

55. Mali, Shrikant. "Anaphylaxis during the Perioperative Period." *Anesthesia: Essays and Researches* 6, no. 2 (2012): 124. https://doi.org/10.4103/0259-1162.108286.

56. Rosenberg, Andrew L., Ronald E. Dechert, Pauline K. Park, and Robert H. Bartlett. "Review of a Large Clinical Series: Association of Cumulative Fluid Balance on Outcome in Acute Lung Injury: A Retrospective Review of the Ardsnet Tidal Volume Study Cohort." *Journal of Intensive Care Medicine* 24, no. 1 (2008): 35–46. https://doi.org/10.1177/0885066608329850.

57. Bhaskar, Priya, Archana V. Dhar, Marita Thompson, Raymond Quigley, and Vinai Modem. "Early Fluid Accumulation in Children with Shock and ICU Mortality: A Matched Case–Control Study." *Intensive Care Medicine* 41, no. 8 (2015): 1445–53. https://doi.org/10.1007/s00134-015-3851-9.

58. Sutherland, Scott M., Michael Zappitelli, Steven R. Alexander, Annabelle N. Chua, Patrick D. Brophy, Timothy E. Bunchman, Richard Hackbarth, et al. "Fluid Overload and Mortality in Children Receiving Continuous Renal Replacement Therapy: The Prospective Pediatric Continuous Renal Replacement Therapy Registry." *American Journal of Kidney Diseases* 55, no. 2 (2010): 316–25. https://doi.org/10.1053/j.ajkd.2009.10.048.

59. Lex, Daniel J., Roland Tóth, Nikoletta R. Czobor, Stephen I. Alexander, Tamás Breuer, Erzsébet Sápi, András Szatmári, Edgár Székely, János Gál, and Andrea Székely. "Fluid Overload Is Associated with Higher Mortality and Morbidity in Pediatric Patients Undergoing Cardiac Surgery*." *Pediatric Critical Care Medicine* 17, no. 4 (2016): 307–14. https://doi.org/10.1097/pcc.0000000000000659.

60. Bion, Julian, Roman Jaeschke, B. Taylor Thompson, Mitchell Levy, and R. Phillip Dellinger. "Surviving Sepsis Campaign: International Guidelines for Management of Severe Sepsis and Septic Shock: 2008." *Intensive Care Medicine* 34, no. 6 (2008): 1163–64. https://doi.org/10.1007/s00134-008-1090-z.

61. Coopersmith, Craig M., Daniel De Backer, Clifford S. Deutschman, Ricard Ferrer, Ishaq Lat, Flavia R. Machado, Greg S. Martin, et al. "Surviving Sepsis Campaign: Research Priorities for Sepsis and Septic Shock." *Intensive Care Medicine* 44, no. 9 (2018): 1400–1426. https://doi.org/10.1007/s00134-018-5175-z.

62. Seymour, Christopher W., Foster Gesten, Hallie C. Prescott, Marcus E. Friedrich, Theodore J. Iwashyna, Gary S. Phillips, Stanley Lemeshow, Tiffany Osborn, Kathleen M. Terry, and Mitchell M. Levy. "Time to Treatment and Mortality during Mandated Emergency Care for Sepsis." *New England Journal of Medicine* 376, no. 23 (2017): 2235–44. https://doi.org/10.1056/nejmoa1703058.

63. Nikolian, Vahagn C., Simone E. Dekker, Ted Bambakidis, Gerald A. Higgins, Isabel S. Dennahy, Patrick E. Georgoff, Aaron M. Williams, Anuska V. Andjelkovic, and Hasan B. Alam. "Improvement of Blood-Brain Barrier Integrity in Traumatic Brain Injury and Hemorrhagic

Shock Following Treatment with Valproic Acid and Fresh Frozen Plasma." *Critical Care Medicine* 46, no. 1 (2018). https://doi.org/10.1097/ccm.0000000000002800.

64. Johansson, Pär I., Jakob Stensballe, Lars S. Rasmussen, and Sisse R. Ostrowski. "A High Admission Syndecan-1 Level, a Marker of Endothelial Glycocalyx Degradation, Is Associated with Inflammation, Protein C Depletion, Fibrinolysis, and Increased Mortality in Trauma Patients." *Annals of Surgery* 254, no. 2 (2011): 194–200. https://doi.org/10.1097/sla.0b013e318226113d.

65. Ostrowski, Sisse Rye, Nicolai Haase, Rasmus Beier Müller, Morten Hylander Møller, Frank Christian Pott, Anders Perner, and Pär Ingemar Johansson. "Association between Biomarkers of Endothelial Injury and Hypocoagulability in Patients with Severe Sepsis: A Prospective Study." *Critical Care* 19, no. 1 (2015). https://doi.org/10.1186/s13054-015-0918-5.

66. Rodriguez, Erika Gonzalez, Sisse R. Ostrowski, Jessica C. Cardenas, Lisa A. Baer, Jeffrey S. Tomasek, Hanne H. Henriksen, Jakob Stensballe, et al. "Syndecan-1: A Quantitative Marker for the Endotheliopathy of Trauma." *Journal of the American College of Surgeons* 225, no. 3 (2017): 419–27. https://doi.org/10.1016/j.jamcollsurg.2017.05.012.

67. Whitney, Jane E., Binqing Zhang, Natalka Koterba, Fang Chen, Jenny Bush, Kathryn Graham, Simon F. Lacey, et al. "Systemic Endothelial Activation Is Associated with Early Acute Respiratory Distress Syndrome in Children with Extrapulmonary Sepsis*." *Critical Care Medicine* 48, no. 3 (2020): 344–52. https://doi.org/10.1097/ccm.0000000000004091.

68. Zeineddin, Ahmad, Jing-Fei Dong, Feng Wu, Pranaya Terse, and Rosemary A. Kozar. "Role of Von Willebrand Factor after Injury: It May Do More than We Think." *Shock* 55, no. 6 (2020): 717–22. https://doi.org/10.1097/shk.0000000000001690.

69. "Dexamethasone in Hospitalized Patients with Covid-19 | Nejm." Accessed March 23, 2023. https://www.nejm.org/doi/full/10.1056/NEJMoa2021436.

70. Norton, Edward C., Morgen M. Miller, and Lawrence C. Kleinman. "Computing Adjusted Risk Ratios and Risk Differences in Stata." *The Stata Journal: Promoting communications on statistics and Stata* 13, no. 3 (2013): 492–509. https://doi.org/10.1177/1536867x1301300304.

71. Barbash, Ian J. "Moving Forward: Frailty and Adverse Sepsis Outcomes*." *Critical Care Medicine* 50, no. 5 (2022): 880–82. https://doi.org/10.1097/ccm.0000000000005377.

72. Rhee, Chanu, Raymund Dantes, Lauren Epstein, David J. Murphy, Christopher W. Seymour, Theodore J. Iwashyna, Sameer S. Kadri, et al. "Incidence and Trends of Sepsis in US Hospitals Using Clinical vs Claims Data, 2009-2014." *JAMA* 318, no. 13 (2017): 1241. https://doi.org/10.1001/jama.2017.13836.

73. Jeremy M. Kahn, MD. "Association between State-Mandated Protocolized Sepsis Care and in-Hospital Adult Sepsis Mortality." JAMA. JAMA Network, July 16, 2019. https://jamanetwork.com/journals/jama/fullarticle/2738290.

74. Coopersmith CM, De Backer D; Deutschman CS, Ferrer R;L Machado FR, Martin GS, Martin-Loeches I. Nunnally ME, Antonelli M, Evans LE, Hellman J. Jog S. Kesecioglu J. Levy MM, Rhodes A; "Surviving Sepsis Campaign: Research Priorities for Sepsis and Septic Shock." Intensive care medicine. U.S. National Library of Medicine. Accessed March 22, 2023. https://pubmed.ncbi.nlm.nih.gov/29971592/.

75. School, 1Division of Graduate. "The Endothelial Glycocalyx: A Fundamental Determinant of Pediatric Critical Care Medicine." LWW. Accessed March 22, 2023. https://journals.lww.com/pccmjournal/Abstract/2020/05000/The_Endothelial_GlycocalyxA_Fundamental.32.aspx.

76. Cao, Rui-Na, Li Tang, Zhong-Yuan Xia, and Rui Xia. "Endothelial Glycocalyx as a Potential Therapeutic Target in Organ Injuries." *Chinese Medical Journal* 132, no. 8 (2019): 963–75. https://doi.org/10.1097/cm9.0000000000000177.

77. Office for Human Research Protections (OHRP). "45 CFR 46." HHS.gov, January 7, 2022. https://www.hhs.gov/ohrp/regulations-and-policy/regulations/45-cfr-46/index.html.

78. Green, Jonathan M., and Holly A. Taylor. "Improving Sepsis Care: Is It Research? Promoting Clarity in a Zone of Confusion*." *Critical Care Medicine* 50, no. 3 (2022): 516–19. https://doi.org/10.1097/ccm.0000000000005279.

79. Kass, Nancy E., and Ruth R. Faden. "Ethics and Learning Health Care: The Essential Roles of Engagement, Transparency, and Accountabili-

ty." *Learning Health Systems* 2, no. 4 (2018). https://doi.org/10.1002/lrh2.10066.

80. Fiest KM, Krewulak KD, Brundin-Mather R, Leia MP, Fox-Robichaud A;Lamontagne F;Leigh, JP 'Patient, Public, and Healthcare Professionals' Sepsis Awareness, Knowledge, and Information Seeking Behaviors: A Scoping Review." Critical Care Medicine. U.S. National Library of Medicine. Accessed March 22, 2023. https://pubmed.ncbi.nlm.nih.gov/35481953/.

81. Pediatrics, 1 Department of. "I Cannot Let It Go: Pediatric Critical Care Medicine." LWW. Accessed March 22, 2023. https://journals.lww.com/pccmjournal/Citation/2022/03000/I_Cannot_Let_It_Go.9.aspx.

82. Belda, Sylvia. "The Unequal Fight." *Pediatric Critical Care Medicine* 23, no. 9 (2022): 745–46. https://doi.org/10.1097/pcc.0000000000003005.

83. Oldner, A., P. Rossi, S. Karason, and A. Åneman. "A Practice Survey on Vasopressor and Inotropic Drug Therapy in Scandinavian Intensive Care Units." *Acta Anaesthesiologica Scandinavica* 47, no. 6 (2003): 693–701. https://doi.org/10.1034/j.1399-6576.2003.00129.x.

84. Klompas M, Rhee C;Singer. "The Importance of Shifting Sepsis Quality Measures from Processes to Outcomes." JAMA. U.S. National Library of Medicine. Accessed March 22, 2023. https://pubmed.ncbi.nlm.nih.gov/36662507/.

This is an abbreviated list of articles used to buttress the contents of the book. These listed articles address the components discussed but are not intended to be inclusive comprehensive references.

The research articles are available to all, using standard search methods. Each individual will benefit maximally when the search is personally performed. The complex subject of sepsis allows the individual to adjust the focus and depth of their interest for optimal results.

All this information is available to the public without restriction.

About the Author

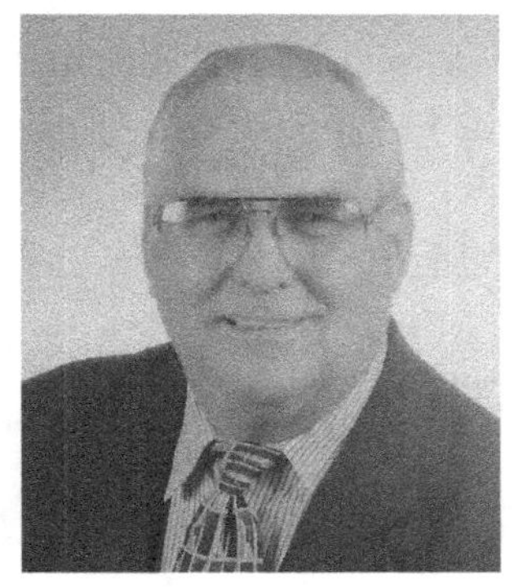

WILLIAM J. NORBERG MD was born to William and Wellma Norberg February 6, 1942, at Moose Lake Minnesota. He grew up on a dairy farm raising Registered Guernsey at Barnum Minnesota. His education was at the small local school. He was involved and successful in all available activities in school and the community.

He attended the University of Minnesota receiving a Bachelor of Science and a Medical Degree. He interned at the University of Kentucky. He practiced General Medicine in Detroit Lakes Minnesota for four years.

He enrolled in the University of Minnesota Pediatric Residency Training Program and upon completion he entered the Pediatric Cardiology Fellowship Program. He received Board Certification in Pediatrics and Pediatric Cardiology following his training. He received Board Certification in the First group of Pediatric Intensivists in that new specialty.

He practiced direct patient care but was always associated with the academic programs in his area.

He had clinical appointments to University of North Dakota, University of Minnesota, University of Texas San Antonio, University of Colorado, University of Southwest Florida, and University of Texas Rio Grande Valley.

He published many journal articles and participated in medical education activities. He directed the rescue of a child who had been under the ice in a river for one hour. This rescue and the patient's intact survival was shown worldwide in 1987. The story became the first 911 Rescue Vignette and is available on YouTube Channel as "The Icy River of the North Rescue 911" He has always been at the forefront of applied techniques in patient care.

He was active in building Pediatric Intensive Care and Children's hospital programs. He was the Medical Director of Children's Hospital Merit-Care in Fargo North Dakota; He was the Medical Director of the Methodist Hospital PICU in San Antonio Texas. He is a member of the Society of Critical Care Medicine, The AMA, and the Academy of Pediatrics and other organizations

He enjoyed his years as one the pioneers in Critical Care Medicine. He is now retired in Florida and writing books and articles about Critical c\Care.

He is particularly proud of his discovery of the breakthrough medical product, TNS that changes the whole focus of the treatments of sepsis.

www.ingramcontent.com/pod-product-compliance
Lightning Source LLC
Chambersburg PA
CBHW071430130726
47997CB00006B/2023